Essentials of Environmental Sciences and Hygiene

for Nursing and Pharmacy Students

Essentials of Environmental Sciences and Hygiene

for Nursing and Pharmacy Students

As per INC Syllabus/PCI (Pharmacy Council of India)

HCL Rawat
Professor and Principal
University College of Nursing
Baba Farid University of Health Sciences
Faridkot, Punjab, India

Satinder Kaur
Faculty
University College of Nursing
Baba Farid University of Health Sciences
Faridkot, Punjab, India

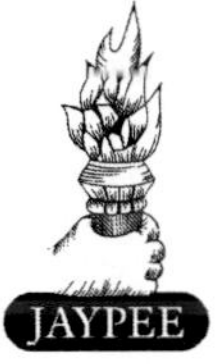

JAYPEE BROTHERS MEDICAL PUBLISHERS
The Health Sciences Publisher
New Delhi | London

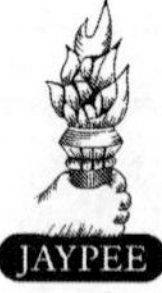

Jaypee Brothers Medical Publishers (P) Ltd

Headquarters
EMCA House
23/23-B, Ansari Road, Daryaganj
New Delhi - 110 002, India
Landline: +91-11-23272143, +91-11-23272703
+91-11-23282021, +91-11-23245672
E-mail: jaypee@jaypeebrothers.com

Corporate Office
4838/24, Ansari Road, Daryaganj
New Delhi - 110 002, India
Phone: +91-11-43574357
Fax: +91-11-43574314
E-mail: jaypee@jaypeebrothers.com

Overseas Office
J.P. Medical Ltd
83 Victoria Street, London
SW1H 0HW (UK)
Phone: +44 20 3170 8910
E-mail: info@jpmedpub.com

EU GPSR Authorised Representative
Logos Europe, 9 rue Nicolas Poussin
17000, La Rochelle, France
Phone: +33 (0) 6 67 93 73 78
E-mail: contact@logoseurope.eu

Website: www.jaypeebrothers.com
Website: www.jaypeedigital.com

Essentials of Environmental Sciences and Hygiene for Nursing and Pharmacy Students

First Edition: **2018**

Reprint: **2026**

ISBN: 978-93-5270-295-4

Printed at: Samrat Offset Pvt. Ltd.

Dedicated to

our beloved parents

Shri Ram Het Rawat
Smt Lahori Devi

Shri Balkar Singh
Smt Amarjit Kaur

Preface

We all live on planet earth, which is the only planet known to have an environment, where air and water are two basic things that sustain life. Without air and water the earth would be like the other planets—no life and no plants.

The environment and environmental protection has been a burning issue for several years in almost every country or globally and time-to-time several steps have been taken by government of various countries to preserve and conserve the environment in the interest of people residing across the globe. There is alarming evidence that important tipping points, leading to irreversible changes in major ecosystems and the planetary climate system, may already have been reached or passed. We are certain beyond a reasonable doubt, however, that the problem of human-caused climate change is real, serious, and immediate, and this problem poses significant risks—to our ability to thrive and build a better future, to national security, to human health and food production and to the interconnected web of living systems.

An essential problem of the 21st century is world pollution. Currently the environment is so contaminated that urgent measures should be taken. A single individual cannot be blamed for the world pollution; however every person should take care of his or her habitat. In addition, it is vital that environmental issues are treated internationally.

This book *Essentials of Environmental Sciences and Hygiene* deals in deep knowledge about different aspects of environment, environmental pollution and health hazards, natural resources and conservation, biodiversity, eco-system, population explosion, current environmental issues and environmental protection measures and at last disaster management.

The nurses and pharmacy students play a vital role in educating people and patients about the importance of environmental hygiene and protection of natural environment. We are sure that this book will prove to be ideal and useful for nursing and pharmacy students to accomplish the objective of acquiring recommended knowledge to qualify examination prescribed by universities. There is always a scope to make improvements and we will try to improve and incorporate suggestions in forthcoming editions.

We, as authors of this book are highly thankful to readers for their valuable suggestions in future.

HCL Rawat
Satinder Kaur

Acknowledgments

A dream does not become reality through magic;
it takes sweat, determination and hard work.

We owe our sincere gratitude and success to God, the Almighty who accompanied and blessed us with his immense grace throughout this project.

It is always difficult to acknowledge so precious a department as that of learning, as it is the only department that is difficult to repay, except through gratitude.

We are extremely grateful to our parents and will always remain obliged for their valuable encouragement and blessings to accomplish this project.

We also owe our sincere gratitude and thanks to our siblings, friends and colleagues for their immense encouragement and interminable support to made this book a success. We appreciate their supportive behavior and comprehensive understanding towards us throughout the project. In all we can say, 'goodness can never be defied and good human being can never be denied.'

We are grateful to Mr Rishi Sourabh Sharma (Associate Director) and Ms Ruby Sharma (Project Manager) of Jaypee Brothers Medical Publishers for giving us an opportunity to develop manuscript related to environmental sciences and hygiene and also to whole staff for publishing this book.

INC Syllabus

ENVIRONMENTAL HYGIENE

Course Description

This course is designed to help students acquire the concept of health, understanding of the principles of environmental health and its relation to nursing in health and disease.

General Objectives

Upon completion of this course, the students shall be able to:

- Describe the concept and principles of environmental health.
- Demonstrate skills to apply the principles of environmental hygiene in caring for self and others.
- Describe the environmental health hazards, related health problems and the services available to meet them.

Total hours: 30

Unit	*Learning objectives*	*Content unit wise*	*Hours*	*Teaching learning activities*	*Method of assessment*	*Chapter*
I	Explain the importance of healthy environment and its relation to health and disease	**Introduction** • Components of environment • Importance of healthy environment	2	Lecture cum discussions	Short answer	1
II	Describe the environmental factors contributing to health and illness	**Environmental factors contributing to health** *Water* • Source and characteristics of safe and wholesome water • Uses of water • Rain water harvesting • Water pollution—natural and acquired impurities • Water borne diseases • Water purification—small and large scale	22	Lecture cum discussions Demonstration Exhibits Visit to water purification plant, sewage treatment plant	Short answer Objective type Essay type	3, 4

Unit	*Learning objectives*	*Content unit wise*	*Hours*	*Teaching learning activities*	*Method of assessment*	*Chapter*
		Air • Composition of air • Airborne diseases • Air pollution and its effect on health • Control of air pollution and use of safety measures *Waste* • Refuse—garbage, excreta and sewage • Health hazards • Waste management: Collection, transportation and disposal *Housing* • Location • Type • Characteristics of good housing • Basic amenities • Town planning *Ventilation* • Types and standards of ventilation *Lighting* • Requirements of good lighting • Natural and artificial lighting • Use of solar energy *Noise* • Sources of noise • Community noise levels • Effects of noise pollution • Noise control measures *Arthropods* • Mosquitoes, housefly, sandfly, human louse, rat fleas, rodents, ticks, etc. • Control measures				4
III	Describe the community organization to promote environmental health	**Community organizations to promote environmental health** *Levels and types of agencies* • National, state, local • Government, voluntary and social agencies *Legislations and acts regulating the environmental hygiene*	6	Lecture cum discussions	Short answer Objective type	7,8,9

PCI
(Pharmacy Council of India)

BPH-108: ENVIRONMENTAL SCIENCES
THEORY

Max. marks: 80 **Total hours: 50 (2 hrs/week)**

S. No.	Content	Chapter
1	**Environmental studies:** Definition, scope and importance. Multidisciplinary nature of environmental studies. *(2)*	1
2.	**Ecosystem:** Structure and functional components of ecosystem. Producers, consumers and decomposers. Food chain and food web. Energy flow and material cycling in ecosystem. Balanced ecosystem. *(3)*	5,7
3.	Environmental pollution: Definition, causes, effects and control measures of water pollution (water quality standards and parameters, assessment of water quality, transformation process in water bodies, oxygen transfer by water bodies, turbulent mixing, water quality in lakes and preservers, groundwater quality), air pollution, soil pollution and noise pollution. *(5)*	1,7,8
4.	**Current environmental issues:** Population growth, human health and urbanization. Global warming (greenhouse effect), climate change, acid rain, ozone layer depletion, industrial and nuclear accidents, nosocomial diseases. *(7)*	6
5.	Environmental protection: Salient features of Environmental Protection Act. Air and Water Acts, Wild life and Forest Acts, functions of central and state pollution control boards. Role of NGO'S, environmental education, role of information technology in environment and human health. *(7)*	2,8,9
6.	**Waste management:** *(8)* • **Water treatment:** Water quality standards, water sources and their quality, water treatment processes, pretreatment of water, conventional process, advanced water treatment process. • **Waste water treatment:** Waterflow rate and characteristics, design of waste water network. Waste water treatment process, pretreatment, primary and secondary treatment of waste water, activated sludge treatment: Anaerobic digestion and its application. • **Solid waste management:** Sources, classification and composition of MSW; properties and separation, storage and transportation, MSW management. Waste minimization, reuse and recycling, biological treatment, thermal treatment, landfill, integrated waste management. Hazardous waste management, hazardous waste and their generation, medical hazardous waste. Household waste, transportation and treatment of hazardous waste: Incinerators, inorganic waste treatment, treatment systems for hazardous waste, handling of treatment plant residue.	2,4

Contents

1. Environment **1**
- Environmental Hygiene *1*
- Environmental Sciences *2*
- Composition of Environment/Types of Environment *4*
- Need of Public Awareness about Environment *7*
- Importance of Healthy Environment *7*

2. Natural Resources **11**
- Natural Resources *11*
- Types of Natural Resources *11*
- Importance of Natural Resources *12*
- Natural Resources and Associated Problems *13*
- Water Resources and Associated Problems *13*
- Mineral Resources *14*
- Food Resources *15*
- Energy Resources *17*

3. Environmental Pollution **21**
- Water Pollution *21*
- Water Conservation and Water Sources Purification *28*
- Waterborne Diseases *29*
- Water Purification *31*
- Air Pollution *36*
- Airborne Disease *40*
- Noise Pollution *41*
- Soil Pollution *43*
- Marine Pollution *45*
- Radioactive Pollution *47*
- Housing and Ventilation *49*
- Ventilation *51*

4. Waste Management **57**
- Waste *57*
- Types of Waste *57*

5. Ecosystem **71**
- Ecology *71*
- Ecosystem *72*
- Introduction and Characteristics of All Types of Ecosystems *82*

6. Current Environmental Issues **88**
- Human Population and Environment *88*
- Human Health and Urbanization *93*
- Acid Rain *95*
- Climate Changes *97*
- Ozone Depletion *98*
- Global Warming *99*

7. Biodiversity: Conservation and Importance **101**
- Biodiversity *101*
- Biodiversity Conservation *103*

8. Environmental Protection **107**
- Environmental Protection Act *107*
- Air (Prevention and Control of Pollution) Act, India *108*
- Water (Prevention and Control of Pollution) Act *109*
- The Forest (Conservation) Act *114*
- Role of NGO's in Environmental Education/ Environmental Protection *114*
- Role of Information Technology in Environment and Human Health *115*

9. Disaster Management **118**
- Disaster *118*
- Disaster Management *119*

Index *125*

CHAPTER 1

Environment

Learning Objectives

At the end of study of this unit students will be able to:

- Define environment and environmental science and hygiene.
- Describe about components of environment.
- Enlist objectives and principles of environmental studies.
- Discuss the scope of environmental studies.
- Define environmental health.
- Discuss importance of environmental health.

■ INTRODUCTION

The term environment has been derived from French word 'Environia' means 'to surround.'

The natural environment encompasses all living and non- living things occur naturally.

The environment encompasses the interaction of all living species, climate, weather and natural resources that affect human survival and economic activity.

■ DEFINITION

The surroundings or conditions in which a person, animal or plant lives or operates.

Or

The natural world, as a whole or in a particular geographical area, especially as affected by human activity.

Or

Environmental Protection Act 1986 defines environment as the sum total of water, air and land, their interrelationships among themselves and with human beings and with other living beings and property.

■ ENVIRONMENTAL HYGIENE

Definition: Environmental hygiene is a group of activities or measures which are undertaken to protect natural environment as well as people from hazardous effects of unsanitary shelter, air and water pollution, industrial and chemical waste, etc.

The aims of environmental hygiene are:

- To maintain and improve standards of basic environmental conditions.
- To provide clean and safe water supply.

- To maintain efficient and safe animal, human, and industrial waste disposal.
- To protect of food from biological and chemical contaminants.
- To maintain adequate housing in clean and safe surroundings.
- To prevent disasters.

ENVIRONMENTAL SCIENCES

Definition: It is an interdisciplinary academic field that integrates physical, biological and information sciences (including ecology, biology, physics, chemistry, zoology, mineralogy, oceanology, limnology, soil science, geology, atmospheric science, and geodesy) to the study of the environment, and the solution of environmental problems. Environmental science emerged from the fields of natural history and medicine during the Enlightenment. Today it provides an integrated, quantitative, and interdisciplinary approach to the study of environmental systems.

Objectives of Environmental Sciences

The need for sustainable development is key point to the future of mankind and survival of universe, thus importance of environmental studies cannot be disputed.

The persistent degradation of ecosystem and environment, i.e. uncontrollable pollution, loss of forests, global warming, depletion of ozone layer, loss of drinkable water etc. threatened to life, economical productivity, and national as well as ecological security. Therefore the environmental studies become necessity in the curriculum to obtain following objectives:

- To develop scientific abilities and understandings consonance with social and environmental concerns.
- To encompass and locate relationship between social, natural and cultural environment.
- To comprehend the complexity of biodiversity.
- To develop a cognitive ability and affect based on observation and illustration based on live experiences and physical, biological, cultural and social aspects of life.
- To nurture curiosity and creativity particularly in relation to natural environment and existence of life, flow of energy and materials in environment.
- To create awareness regarding various environmental issues like biodegradation, global warming, natural threats to life, etc.
- To understand various biotic and abiotic components of environment.
- To help social groups and individuals to acquire a set of values for environmental protection.

Principles of Environmental Sciences

- To foster clear awareness and concern about economic, social, political and ecological interdependence in urban and rural areas.
- To create new patterns of behaviors of individuals, groups and society as a whole towards the environment.

- To provide every person with opportunities to acquire the knowledge, values, attitudes, commitment and skills needed to protect and improve the environment.

According to UNESCO, the guiding principles of environmental education should be as follows:

- Environmental education should be compulsory, right from the primary up to the postgraduate stage.
- Environmental education should have an interdisciplinary approach by including physical, chemical, biological as well as sociocultural aspects of the environment. It should build a bridge between biology and technology.
- Environmental education should take into account the historical perspective, the current and the potential historical issues.
- Environmental education should emphasize the importance of sustainable development, i.e. economic development without degrading the environment.
- Environmental education should emphasize the necessity of seeking international cooperation in environmental planning.
- Environmental education should lay more stress on practical activities and first hand experiences.

Scope and Importance of Environmental Sciences

The disciplines included in environmental education are environmental sciences, environmental engineering and environmental management.

- ***Environmental science:*** It deals with the scientific study of environmental system (air, water, soil and land), the inherent or induced changes on organisms and the environmental damages incurred as a result of human interaction with the environment
- ***Environmental engineering:*** It deals with the study of technical processes involved in the protection of environment from the potentially deleterious effects of human activity and improving the environmental quality for the health and well-beings of humans.
- ***Environmental management:*** It promotes due regard for physical, social and economic environment of the enterprise or projects. It encourages planned investment at the start of the production chain rather than forced investment in cleaning up at the end.

  It generally covers the areas as environment and enterprise objectives, scope, and structure of the environment, interaction of nature, society and the enterprise, environment impact assessment, economics of pollution, prevention, environmental management standards, etc.
- ***Environmental studies and environmental pollution control:*** The knowledge of environmental sciences contributes to pollution control to great extent. It has great scope in pollution control departments like person can be appointed as an assistant environmental officers, environmental officer in pollution control board, industries, sewage treatment plants after graduation and postgraduation in environmental sciences. One can start his own environmental pollution control consultancy and can

contribute in research work related to environmental pollution control as well as can join as lecturers in educational institutes and universities to teach environmental sciences.

Importance of Environmental Sciences

The importance of environmental studies is as follows:

- To clarify modern environmental concept like how to conserve biodiversity.
- To know the more sustainable way of living.
- To use natural resources more efficiently.
- To know the behavior of organism under natural conditions.
- To know the interrelationship between organisms in populations and communities.
- To aware and educate people regarding environmental issues and problems at local, national and international levels.

■ COMPOSITION OF ENVIRONMENT/TYPES OF ENVIRONMENT

The major components of environment include atmosphere, hydrosphere, lithosphere and biosphere.

But as per immediate categorization of environments components are:

- ***Microenvironment/socioculture environment:*** Microenvironment refers to immediate local surroundings of person, e.g. home, family, work environment. Whereas, socioculture environment is person's society, type of family rituals, beliefs, customs and behavior of person. Sociocultural environment consists of factors related to human relationships and the impact of social attitudes and cultural values on the work of person.
- ***Macro environment/biological and psychological environment:*** Macro environment includes the uncontrollable factors or physical conditions and their impact on person as well as external factors which put impact on health and work of person, e.g. area of interest, job satisfaction, stresses level and coping, health status, etc.
- ***Physical environment:*** Physical environment is a geographic environment which includes all external natural environment conditions like lightening, air, temperature, rainfall, soil, etc. It influences development of life and human experiences.
- ***Biotic environment:*** Biotic environment includes all things which are living in nature in ecosystem, e.g. plants, microbes, fungi, animals, etc. These living organisms interact with each other and with a biotic environment. This type of environment also includes a number of interrelated populations of same species live in common environment. Biotic factor of environment needs food and energy to survive. It can be categorized into three types:
  1. ***Producers:*** These are organisms that synthesize organic substances. Example: Plants.
  2. ***Consumers:*** Consumers are the organisms that feed on other organisms. Consumers are of three trophic levels depending on the level and

category of their food; they are primary consumer are herbivorous which feeds on plants and fungus, e.g. cattles., secondary consumers are carnivorous which prey on other animals, e.g. lion and tertiary consumers are omnivorous which feeds on both plants and animals, e.g. humans.

3. ***Decomposers:*** These are saprophytes—microorganisms that feed on dead and decayed waste matter. Examples: Bacteria and fungi.

Environment is the sum total of conditions that surrounds us at a given point of time and space. It is comprised of the interacting systems of physical, biological and cultural elements which are interlinked both individually and collectively. Environment is the sum total of conditions in which an organism has to survive or maintain its life process. It influences the growth and development of living forms. Thus, environment refers to anything that is immediately surrounding an object and exerting a direct influence on it.

Environment comprises of various components. Except discussed earlier there are certain important components of environment which influences universe. These are as follows:

Physical Components

The most important physical components of environment are as follows:

Biosphere

Biosphere refers to realm of living organisms and their interaction with environment (atmosphere, hydrosphere and lithosphere).

Biosphere is very large and complex system made up of smaller units known as ecosystem.

Ecosystem composed of physical factors such as soil, water and air constitute ecosystem which is definite zone for plants, animals and micro-organisms to live.

Atmosphere

Atmosphere plays vital role in survival of earth planet

- ***Protective blanket:*** It is composed of gases which protect earth from hostile environment of space.
- ***Absorption:*** It absorbs and reemits infrared rays from earth and maintains temperature of earth.
- ***Transmission:*** It allows transmission of radiation and filters tissue damaging UV rays
- ***Photosynthesis:*** Act as source of CO_2 to enhance photosynthesis and helps in producing O_2 in environment.
- ***Nitrogen source:*** Act a source of nitrogen for nitrogen fixing bacteria & ammonia producing plants.
- **Transportation:** Atmosphere transport water from ocean to land.

Atmospheric Components

Atmosphere: Atmosphere surrounds the dangerous rays from sun. The atmosphere composed of mixture of gases (e.g. CO_2, O_2, NO_2 etc.)

Atmosphere has five layers:

1. ***Troposphere:*** Troposphere is first layer above the surface. Weather is a part of this layer.
2. ***Stratosphere:*** This is a stable layer which contains ozone helps in absorbing harmful rays of sun.
3. ***Mesosphere:*** Composed of meteors or rock fragments.
4. ***Thermosphere:*** This is a layer with auroras. This is a layer where space shuttle orbits.
5. ***Exosphere:*** This is upper limit of atmosphere where it merges with space.

Hydrosphere

Collective term used for all different forms of water. This is the term which includes all types of water resources such as ocean, sea, rivers, lakes, streams, reservoirs, glaciers and groundwater.

The distribution of earth's water supply is shown in Figure 1.1.

Lithosphere

It includes composition of earth. Earth has main three layers as shown in Figure 1.2.

Lithosphere consists of mantle, crust and inner and outer core. Crust is outer skin of earth composed of rocks and soil which is accessible to humans.

Components of Earth

- ***Equator:*** Equator is an imaginary line on the earth's surface equidistant from north pole and south pole that divides the earth into a northern hemisphere and a southern hemisphere.
- ***Altitude:*** Altitude is a distance measurement usually in the vertical or 'up' direction between a reference datum and a point or object.

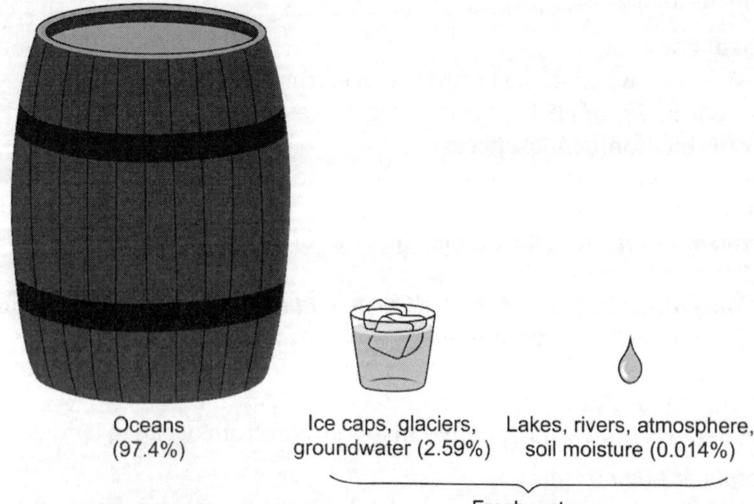

Fig. 1.1: Distribution of earth's water supply

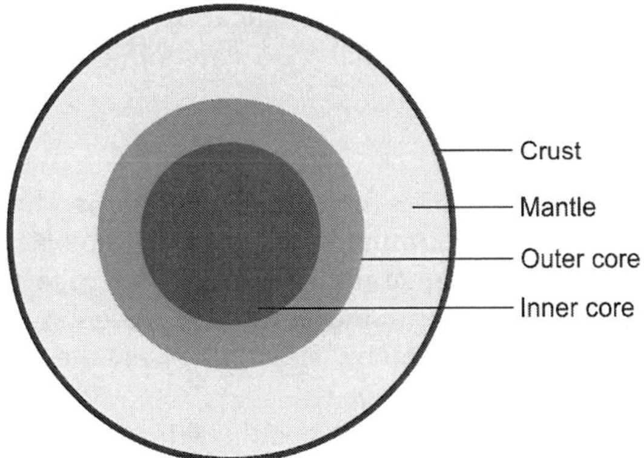

Fig. 1.2: Layers of the earth

NEED OF PUBLIC AWARENESS ABOUT ENVIRONMENT

In today's world because of industrialization and increasing population, the natural resources has been rapidly utilized and our environment is being increasingly degraded by human activities, so we need to protect the environment.

It is not only the duty of government but also the people to take active role for protecting the environment, so protecting our environment is economically more viable than cleaning it up once, it is damaged.

The role of mass media such as newspapers, radio, television, etc is also very important to make people aware regarding environment. There are various institutions, which are playing positive role towards environment to make people aware regarding environment like BSI (Botanical Survey of India, 1890), ZSI (Zoological Survey of India, 1916), WII (Wild Life Institute of India, 1982) etc.

IMPORTANCE OF HEALTHY ENVIRONMENT

Environmental health comprises those aspects of human health, including quality of life, that are determined by physical, biological, social, and psychosocial factors in the environment. It also refers to the theory and practice of assessing, correcting, controlling, and preventing those factors in the environment that can potentially affect adversely the health of present and future generations.

Definition of Health

A state of complete physical, mental, and social well-being and not merely the absence of disease or infirmity (WHO, 1948).

Definition of Environment

Environment is the circumstance, objects or conditions by which one is surrounded.

It can be divided into physical, biological, social, and cultural factors and anything external to individual who can influence health status in populations.

Environmental Health

Environmental health comprises those aspects of human health, including quality of life, that are determined by physical, biological, social, and psychosocial factors in the environment. It also refers to the theory and practice of assessing, correcting, controlling, and preventing those factors in the environment that can potentially affect adversely the health of present and future generations.

Environment can be considered as healthy when it has zero risk of harm and is free from threat of danger, harm, injury or illness and loss to any living organism.

To maintain healthy environment and create awareness the world environment day is celebrated every year on 5th, June.

Importance of Healthy Environment

The human activities are creating consequences to harm healthy environment for all kingdoms (animal and plant). The industry and emission of carbon in tons on daily basis is putting a significant adverse effect on human as well as natural habitat.

The individual, society and environment all these are interdependent to each other as shown in Figure 1.3.

Thus, as human and society actions put effect on each other, environment reverses these effects too.

Therefore, healthy environment is needed for healthy body and sound mind.

Thus this is great demand of present to take efforts to save and restore healthy environment to prevent destructive consequences in future life.

- Living in green and healthy surroundings lowers blood pressure, improve attention and immunity.
- The decrease in global warming and emissions from human fossil fuels will decrease temperature of environment results in reduction of natural disasters, heat strokes, malnutrition and will prevent malaria.

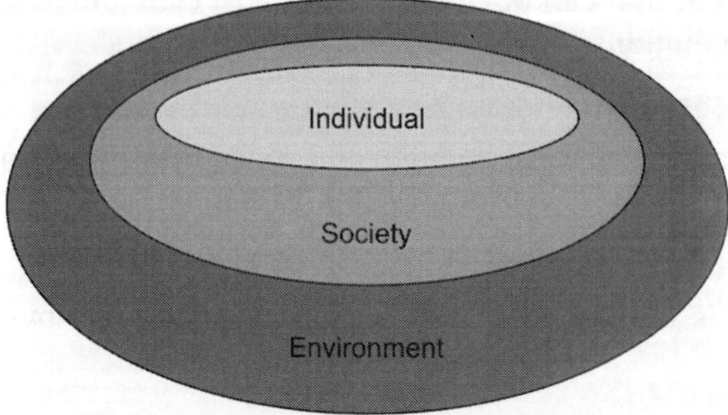

Fig. 1.3: Individual, society and environment

- The decrease in air toxics will reduce incidence of cancer, neurological, reproductive and respiratory system disorders.
- The maintenance of natural water contents and resources will reduce risk of health consequences like gastrointestinal disorders, cancer nervous system and reproductive system disorders.

The present time is in great demand of healthy environment for all living organisms.

Objectives of Environmental Health

The Healthy People 2020 Environmental Health objectives focus on following themes, each of which highlights an element of environmental health:

- Outdoor air quality
- Surface and ground water quality
- Toxic substances and hazardous wastes
- Homes and communities
- Infrastructure and surveillance
- Global environmental health

Outdoor air quality: Poor air quality is linked to premature death, cancer, and long-term damage to respiratory and cardiovascular systems. Progress has been made to reduce unhealthy air emissions. Decreasing air pollution is an important step in creating a healthy environment.

Surface and ground water: Surface and ground water quality applies to both drinking water and recreational waters. Protecting water sources and minimizing exposure to contaminated water sources are important parts of environmental health.

Toxic substances and hazardous wastes: The health effects of toxic substances and hazardous wastes are not yet fully understood. Research to better understand how these exposures may impact health is ongoing. Meanwhile, efforts to reduce exposures continue. Reducing exposure to toxic substances and hazardous wastes is fundamental to environmental health.

Communities and homes: People spend most of their time at home, work or school. Thus it is important to improve indoor air quality by reducing smoking (active and passive), home air filters use and by maintaining cleanliness at home. By encouraging body art safety like to say 'No' to tattooing, piercing of body parts, etc. Accurate food preservation handling and pesticide free production of food particles. We can keep our home and community environment healthy by maintaining housing standard and proper disposal of waste as per recommendations of municipality.

ASSESSMENT

Essay Type Questions

1. Define environment. Describe in detail about components of environment.
2. What do you mean by environmental sciences? Discuss in brief scope and importance of environmental science.

Short Answer Type Questions

1. Define environment health.
2. Write in short about components of earth.
3. Enlist layers of earth.
4. Write principles of environmental sciences.
5. Describe in short about effects of environment on health.

Multiple Choice Questions

1. The blanket of gases surrounds the earth is called:
   (a) Atmosphere (b) Hydrosphere
   (c) Lithosphere (d) Biosphere
2. The collective term used for all sources of water present on earth is:
   (a) Biosphere (b) Hydrosphere
   (c) Lithosphere (d) Atmosphere
3. The surroundings in which any person, plant and organism survive is called:
   (a) Environment (b) Society
   (c) Home (d) Universe
4. The environment in which all living things are included is:
   (a) Physical environment (b) Biotic environment
   (c) Macro environment (d) Microenvironment
5. The organisms which feed on other organisms are called:
   (a) Producers (b) Decomposers
   (c) Consumers (d) None of these
6. The World Environment Day is celebrated on:
   (a) 5 June (b) 5 October
   (c) 5 September (d) 5 July

ANSWERS

1. (a) 2. (b) 3. (a) 4. (b)
5. (c) 6. (a)

CHAPTER

2 Natural Resources

Learning Objectives

At the end, students will be able to:
- Define natural resources.
- Describe and classify types of natural resources.
- Understand importance of natural resources.
- Describe associated problems of different types of natural resources.

NATURAL RESOURCES

Introduction

Since the Earth was inhabited, humans and other life forms have depended on things that exist freely in nature to survive can be termed as natural resources and are basis of life on earth. Natural resources can be used directly or indirectly.

A natural resource term refers to material which come from natural environment and people can use to them. For example, air, water, fossil fuels, wood, wild life energy, minerals, etc.

Definition

A material source of wealth such as timber, fresh water or mineral deposit that occurs in a natural state and has an economic value.

Or

Natural resource is something such as forest, mineral deposit or fresh water that is found in nature and is necessary or useful to humans.

Raw Material

Most of the time natural resources are used as a raw or basic material to produce something. For instance, to obtain wood for furniture we take it from trees. Thus, tree is a raw material.

TYPES OF NATURAL RESOURCES

All natural resources on broadways can be categorized into two parts:
1. Renewable resources
2. Non renewable resources

Renewable Resources

The natural resources coined as renewable those are constantly available at earth, and can be replaced or recovered as per need, e.g. water, vegetative land, etc.

Animals are also considered as renewable in nature because replace older with younger through reproduction.

Renewable resources are of two types:

1. ***Organic renewable:*** The raw material which comes from living things like trees, animals, etc. are considered as organic renewable resources.
2. ***Inorganic renewable:*** If material comes from non-living things, e.g. water, soil, air, sun, etc. considered as inorganic renewable resources.

Nonrenewable Resources

The materials or things which cannot be easily replaced or renewed which once destroyed are called non renewable resources, e.g. fossil fuels, minerals, etc.

The process of formation or production of non renewable resource is called rock cycle which takes thousands of years to produce non renewable materials.

Types of Nonrenewable Resources

1. ***Metallic:*** Metallic minerals are those which contain metals. They can be characterized as shiny, harder and melted with heat to produce new things, e.g. iron, copper and tin, etc.
2. ***Non-metallic:*** These minerals do not have any sort of metal in them. Thus, they are softer and non shiny, e.g. clay and coal.

■ IMPORTANCE OF NATURAL RESOURCES

The mankind use natural resources in various forms and are important for development of country. The humans use natural resources in various forms which are as follows:

Food and Drink

The natural resources form agriculture, fresh water, sea, plants, and rocks, which are important in manufacturing of various foods for living organisms specifically for humans.

Agriculture gives us cereals as well as food for animals. The forests give us raw material for food and beverages as well as various plants and shrubs needed in manufacturing of drugs and medicines. The sea and fresh water resources also give us raw material for food rich in minerals and proteins like sea shell, fish, etc.

Mobility

The fossil fuels, petroleum, oil, etc. are required for transportation of automobiles which is provided by natural resources directly or indirectly.

Housing and Infrastructures

The construction material for all sorts of buildings, houses, and roads come from natural resources like rocks, etc.

Basic Needs

Besides materialistic things of our daily living needs like respiration, fresh oxygen, food, drinking water, maintaninence of temperature, etc. all are fulfilled by natural resources.

NATURAL RESOURCES AND ASSOCIATED PROBLEMS

Forest Resources

Forests are home of natural resources and are more blessing for humans. Forests provide us various natural resources which are as follows:

- ***Wood:*** Forests are huge source of wood which can be used as multipurpose. For example, cooking, fire, making shelter, etc.
- ***Timber wood:*** Shelter is a basic need of humans. Thus, forests provide us timber wood needed in construction of house, furniture, in day-to-day life, necessity of tools for agriculture and others.
- ***Foods:*** Forests provide new material for manufacturing of various vegetarian and non-vegetarian foods for humans and animals, e.g. honey, meat, etc.
- ***Shelter:*** A large number of species of animals, birds, microorganisms are provided shelter by forests.
- ***Paper:*** Paper is an important stationary in modern era and raw material in making paper is wood, bamboo and grass which are provided by the forest.
- ***Medicines:*** Forests are the hub of various plants and shrubs those have significant medicinal quality and are needed as a raw material for preparation of various drugs to treat as well as prevent diseases.

Problems Associated with Natural Resources of Forests

- ***Deforestation:*** The continuous cutting of trees and cultivation of forests to convert into residential and commercial area, which is producing major problems in abundance of natural resources like fresh air, wood, water resources, plants, etc. Thus, it is putting great impact on climate conditions as well as increasing global warming on planet.
- ***Timber extraction:*** Timber or wood cultivation from forests for construction of buildings is halting to biodiversity as well as destroying shelter for various birds, insects and animals. They have reduced number of live plants on earth which is causing natural disasters as well as increase in temperature which will lead to unfavorable for maintenance of life on planet.
- ***Mining:*** Mining is the process of extraction of minerals and other valuable metals from earth. It causes emission of suspended particles and gases which causes air pollution. The release of harmful trace elements like Co, Cd, etc. lead to contamination of surface water and seepage of material from mining into soil which causes pollution of groundwater and results in harm to natural flora and fauna.

WATER RESOURCES AND ASSOCIATED PROBLEMS

Water itself is an important natural resource on earth as well as major component in maintenance of life on earth.

It has various uses which are as follows:

- ***Domestic:*** In human life, water is a natural element in every task of daily routine like washing, drinking, cooking, and bathing, etc.

- ***Commercial:*** Water is a raw material almost for every industry and is basic component in preparation of products in various factories like medicines, bakery, hotels, restaurants, fertilizers, various packet food preparations, etc.
- ***Hydropower:*** Water is a basic component in production of electricity by conversion of thermo energy to enlighten human life.
- ***Navigation:*** Water resources like lakes, oceans and rivers are major pathways for national and international trading and import and export of material thus contributing in economical development of country.
- ***Habitat:*** Water resources are natural habitat for various animal and plant species.
- ***Food:*** Water is a major source of sea food and food source for various birds and animals like fish.
- ***Ecosystem:*** Through hydrologic cycle water maintains climate temperature and moisture as well as rainfall table on planet.

Problems Associated with Water Resources

- ***Overutilization:*** Due to population explosion, the increased demand of water is causing scarcity of water resources on earth. To compensate with this problem, Indian Government has taken initiatives for interlinking of rivers in India. For example, the ministry of water resources, Government of India has launched a project to interlink the main Ganga and Brahmaputra to divert their overflow in west.
- ***Water pollution:*** The mixing of harmful and non harmful pollutants in surface and ground water causing the various water resources in unusable form.
- ***Dams:*** Although dams are constructed to a year round supply of water for domestic use for humans but it diverts the natural flow of rivers resulting in floods and deforestation as well as cause harm to wet lands and flood plains. This result in loss of economical things and lives.
- ***Acid rain:*** The pollution of water and mixing of chemicals from agricultural fields as well as industries in surface water results in evaporation of pollulated water as well as later on during condensation certain harmful contents also mix in water from air thus result in acid rain and that causes harm to normal life pattern of ecosystem.
- ***Climate change:*** Due to overutilization of water and increased global warming causing early melting of glaciers which results in disasters and changes in climate of earth.
- ***Droughts:*** Due to increased demand of utilization, deforestation and reduced table of ground water and rain causing scarcity of water resources in various areas of earth resulting in droughts and converting land into deserts.

■ MINERAL RESOURCES

A mineral is an organic substance occurs naturally in the earth's crust which extracts through mining.

Mineral resources can be categorized into three parts:
1. Fuel minerals
2. Metallic minerals
3. Non-metallic minerals

Fuel Minerals

Fuel minerals involve coal, oils and natural gas.

- ***Coal:*** Coal consumption as fuel occurs in both domestic and industrial use. The preparation of coal under earth's surface taken or long periods of years. The increased industrial sectors have increased demand of coal and day-by-day the amount of coal is decreasing in natural part.
- ***Crude oil (petroleum):*** It is believed that petroleum has over a period of millions of years by conversion of fossils into hydrocarbon by heat, pressure and catalytic action. The petroleum is a major product in transporting trough automobiles as well as used by products in various industries.
- ***Natural gas:*** A natural gas is used in domestic and industries for various purposes.

Metallic Minerals

Metallic minerals are hard substances that conduct heat and electricity and have a characteristic luster or shine, e.g. Iron ore, bauxite, manganese ore, etc. have various uses in industry, domestic and health department as well as in construction.

Non-metallic Minerals

Non-metallic minerals do not contain metals, e.g. limestone, salt, mica, potash, nitrates. The minerals fuels like coal and petroleum are also non-metallic minerals.

Mineral Resources and Associated Problems

- ***Hazards of mining:*** Mining is a hazardous procedure for the health of humans. It causes various diseases related to respiratory as well as cardiovascular system among workers of mines.
- ***Rapid depletion of high grade minerals:*** The mining process and extraction of minerals from earth's surface cause erosion of soil as well as causes extraction of minerals and waste material during process causing air and water pollution.
- ***Wastage of upper soil layer and vegetation:*** During extraction of minerals, the erosion of upper soil layer occur which causes destruction of vegetative layer of earth and spread various pollutants in air and mixing of pollutants in surface water resources.
- ***Consumption of energy resources:*** Mining involves huge consumption of energy resources like coal, petroleum, natural gas which are non-renewable resources.

■ FOOD RESOURCES

Food is a basic need of human as well as animal life. Humans consume various types of food. There are three major food resources:

1. ***The croplands:*** The croplands are major resources of food for humans. There are 4 major essential crops which account for caloric consumption of human beings, e.g. potatoes, rice, wheat, and corn.
2. ***The rangelands:*** The rangelands which provide a different source of milk and meat from animals grazing, e.g. goats, cattle and sheep.
3. ***The fisheries:*** The fisheries provide fish which are a major source of animal protein.

Types of Food Production Resources

- ***Industrialized agricultural food resources:*** This is known as high input agricultural and modern farming. This refers to the industrial production of livestock, poultry, fish, and crops. This type of agriculture includes innovation in agricultural mechanisms, genetic technology, techniques for achieving economies of scale in production and global trade, etc.
- ***Traditional agriculture:*** Traditional agriculture is the most widely used method of developing countries. The subsistence agriculture practices only animals and humans labor and produce food only to meet for farmer's family needs.

Problems Associated with Food Resources

Overgrazing

Due to population explosion, a huge population needs to be fed and grazing lands or pasture areas are not adequate. Overgrazing causes problems which are as follows:

- ***Soil erosion:*** Because of overgrazing, the vegetation layer of land gets destroyed. When the grassroots are removed from the upper layer of the soil, it becomes loose and susceptible to the aviation of wind and water.
- ***Land degradation:***
  - Due to loosening of vegetative layer of the soil because of overgrazing, the soil surface lost its structure, hydraulic conductivity and soil becomes susceptible to aviation of wind and water.
  - The soil becomes poor and dry and loses its infiltration capacity resulting in reduction of power of production of water into the soil.
  - Organic cycling also gets impaired due to lack of detritus on the soil to be decomposed.
- ***Loss of useful species:*** Overgrazing adversely affects the biodiversity of plants and their regeneration capacity.
- ***Floods:*** Soil becomes unable to check the flow of rain water and that causes floods. The areas like Assam, West Bengal, Odisha, Andhra Pradesh, Uttar Pradesh, and Punjab are flood prone areas of India during monsoon rain which cause overflow in Ganga, Yamuna and Brahmaputra rivers.

Adverse Impact of Agriculture on Food Resources

- ***Local changes:*** The effects which occur at the site of farming. It brought following changes:
  - Soil erosion
  - Pollution of rivers from fertilizers

- Poisoning of fish due to water pollution
- Depletion of nutrients due to slash and burning of organic matter in soil which destroyed the nutrients.

- ***Regional changes:*** Refers to change in region of farming which are as follows:
  - Deforestation
  - Desertification
  - Soil infertility
  - Large population.
- ***Global changes:*** Changes occur around the world.
  - ***Climatic changes:*** Changes occur in the climate around the world.
  - ***Global warming:*** Due to deforestation, the CO_2 concentration increases in atmosphere which causes increase in temperature.

Effects of Modern Agriculture on Food Resources

- ***Effects related to high-yielding varieties:*** This encourages monocrop and genotype those leads to devastation of crop by disease caused due to pathogens attack and rapid spread of disease.
- ***Water logging:*** The area where tube well water and canal are extensively used by farmers leads to water logging.
- ***Salinity problems:*** Due to excessive irrigation and use of carbonate and bicarbonate of sodium leads to increase in pH of soil causes salinity of soil.

Fertilizers Related Problems

- ***Micronutrient imbalance:*** The excessive use of chemical fertilizers like Nitrogen (N), Phosphorus (P) and Potassium (K) these reduces micro-nutrients in vegetative soil.
- ***Nitrate pollution:*** The nitrogenous fertilizers used on soil seeped down into the ground water and causes water pollution.
- ***Eutrophication:*** Due to mixing of nitrogen, potassium in water resources with runoff water from crop fields causing algae blooming and toxins productions which effect the aquatic food chain.

Pesticide Related Problems

The excessive use of pesticides in fields causes following problems:

- Creating resistance in pests which destroy crops and food chains which are known as 'super pests'.
- ***Biological magnification:*** The excessive use causes accumulation of pesticides in food chain called biological magnification which is hazardous for human population.
- ***Death of useful organisms:*** Due to use of insecticides sometimes favorable organisms also become target.

■ ENERGY RESOURCES

Energy is an important component of basic life process and is the capacity of doing work. The substances which produce energy for utilization to increase work capacity are known as energy resources, e.g. sun, wind, coal, and petroleum, etc. Energy resources can be classified into two types: Non-renewable resources and renewable resources.

Non-renewable Resources

These are also known as conventional resources which are exhaustible and cannot be replaced easily when they are once used. These are fossil fuels, for example, coal, petroleum and natural gas.

Fossil Fuels

- ***Coal:*** Coal is known as prime source of energy. It is an essential material which is used in metallurgical and chemical industries. It is composed of volatile matter, moisture and carbon besides ash content. In India, the major resources of coal are Bihar, West Bengal, Madhya Pradesh, Odisha, Andhra Pradesh, and Maharashtra.
- ***Petroleum and oil:*** Petroleum is an inflammable liquid formed by hydro-carbons, oxygen, nitrogen, sulfur and traces of organ metallic compounds.

  The use of petroleum and petroleum products is mainly for motive power, lubricating agents, and as a raw material in various chemical industries. The major reserves of oil in India are Assam, Gujarat, Mumbai, and Rajasthan.
- ***Natural gas:*** Natural gas found alone or in conjunction with crude oil. It is a major source of energy for thermal power and also used as raw material in petrochemical industry. It helps in building fertilizer plants for agriculture. The major reserves are Assam, Gujarat and Mumbai.

Renewable Resources

These are also known as non-conventional resources. These are never run out resources of energy which exists freely in nature. These are solar energy, wind, water, and biomass.

- ***Biomass:*** Biomass is energy produced by conversion of organic matter or waste like wood, plant, matter, etc. Biomass may be directly used as fuel on processed into liquids and gases. It is cheap and clean source of energy to improve sanitation and hygiene. It also produces enriched organic manure which is used in agriculture.
- ***Wind power:*** The wind energy is produced by huge convection currents in the earth's atmosphere driven by heat energy from the sun. Actually, this is wind's kinetic energy which is transformed into electrical energy using wind turbines. The largest wind turbine in the world is located in Hawaii.
- ***Water energy:*** The kinetic energy of moving water can be transferred into useful energy in various ways. By constructing the dams, the gravitational potential energy is converted into Hydroelectric Power (HEP) with the help of generator. Hydropower does not cause global warming.
- ***Geothermal energy:*** It is the heat energy produced in earth's crust by molten rocks (magma) and this increased the temperature of surface water and rock which can be used to generate power. The best example of this is India is Narmada-son-valley and Damodar valley.

- ***Solar energy:*** Sun is a natural source of solar energy and is freely available in environment.
  - The major use of solar energy is conversion into electricity.
  - Solar energy is stored into different devices to convert their functioning, e.g. solar ponds.
- ***Marine (ocean) energy:*** The ocean has huge potential and resource of power and energy. Marine energy has two potentials:
  1. ***Wave energy:*** When sun strikes at surface of ocean it increased pressure inside water and produces wind which causes waves having kinetic energy and that is stored by wave devices by three means:
     a. ***Point absorber:*** This is a floating structure that moves up and down with waves and converts kinetic energy of waves into power and stored it.
     b. ***The attenuator:*** This device is like wings of bird and floats on surface of ocean and rides the waves. This is also stored kinetic energy of waves as power.
     c. ***The oscillating wave surge converter:*** This device is instilled below the water surface there it extracts energy from waves and stores it.
  2. ***Tidal energy:*** The combination power of sun, moon and gravitational force of earth produce tides in ocean. The tidal kinetic energy is converted into power with the help of horizontal turbines.

Nuclear Energy

Nuclear power is the largest source of electricity in India. Nuclear energy is produced during nuclear fission when uranium rod is used as fuel to produce heat. During this process CO_2 gas and water is pumped through the reactor and produces steam. This steam strikes with turbines and converted into electric power. India has single nuclear plant situated in Kudankulam in state of Tamil Nadu.

ASSESSMENT

Essay Type Questions

1. Define natural resources. Describe in detail about types of natural resources.
2. Describe importance of natural resources. Discuss in detail regarding associated problems of water and energy resources.
3. Define mineral resources and associated problems of mineral resources.

Short Answer Type Questions

1. Define biomass.
2. Describe in brief about wave energy storage.
3. What is nuclear energy?

Multiple Choice Questions

1. Deforestation is term used for:
   (a) Cultivation of forests (b) Vegetation of trees
   (c) Natural forest resources (d) Drought and soil erosion
2. The process of extraction of minerals from earth's surface is known as:
   (a) Mining (b) Soil erosion
   (c) Deforestation (d) None of the above
3. The major resources of food for humans are:
   (a) The rangelands (b) The croplands
   (c) The fisheries (d) None of the above
4. The destruction of upper layer of earth is known as:
   (a) Land degradation (b) Deforestation
   (c) Soil erosion (d) None of the above
5. The mixing of nitrogen and potassium in water resources from crop fields is known as:
   (a) Nitrate pollution (b) Salinity of water
   (c) Eutrophication (d) None of the above

ANSWERS

1. (a) 2. (a) 3. (b) 4. (c)
5. (c)

CHAPTER

Environmental Pollution 3

Learning Objectives

After study this unit students will be able to:

- Define water and sources of water.
- Discuss water pollution and control of water pollution.
- Discuss waterborne diseases and prevention.
- Describe various methods of water harvesting.
- Define air and composition of air.
- Describe air pollution and its ill effects on health.
- Give detail about management of air pollution.
- Enlist diseases caused by air pollution.
- Define noise.
- Describe sources of noise.
- Define noise pollution.
- Enumerate effects on human health of noise pollution.
- Describe about control measures of noise pollution.
- Define soil pollution.
- Describe causes and types of soil pollution.
- Explain different control measures for soil pollution.
- Define marine and marine pollution.
- Describe causes and effects of marine pollution.
- Describe control measures of marine pollution.
- Define radioactivity and radioactive pollution.
- Enlist sources of radioactive pollution
- Describe causes of radioactive pollution.
- Describe effects of radioactive pollution.
- Enumerate control measures of radioactive pollution.
- Define housing.
- Describe housing standards and accurate location for housing.
- Describe construction of healthy house.
- Define ventilation.
- Enumerate type of ventilation.

WATER POLLUTION

Water is a transparent and nearly colorless chemical substance with chemical formula H_2O and is the main constituent of earth's streams, lakes, and oceans, and the fluids of most living organisms. Water strictly refers to the liquid state of that substance, that prevails at standard ambient temperature and pressure but it is also abundant in solid form as ice and gaseous form as vapors. In natural state it occurs as snow, glaciers, clouds, fog dew, etc. in solid and gaseous form.

Definition

Water is a colorless, odorless and tasteless liquid, which plays vital role in animal and human life. This is important solvent to maintain normal physiological processes of life.

Major Physical Characteristics of Water

- Water is non-expensive and easily available molecule
- Water is a polar molecule
- Water can form hydrogen bond with other polar compound
- Freezing point of water is 0°C (32°F)
- Boiling point of water is 100°C
- Normal specific gravity of water is 1.0000 (4°C).

Sources of Water

Life is possible on earth due to the presence of water. Nearly three-fourths of the earth's surface is covered with water. About 70% of the human body is water. The bodies of all plants and animals contain water. Thus water is available in natural sources and manmade sources on earth like—rainwater, oceans, rivers, lakes, streams, ponds and springs are natural sources of water whereas wells, dams, hand pumps, canals etc. are manmade sources of water.

Rainwater

Rainwater collects on the earth in the form of surface water which is present on the surface of earth in oceans, rivers, lakes and underground water is present below soil and rocks. Basically underground water is the rainwater which seeped through soil and collects under the surface which can be obtained by digging wells, sinking tubes and through springs. The collection of rainwater is known as rainwater harvesting. On the surface of earth 94% of water is in oceans and 4% covered by groundwater whereas rivers and other sources cover < 0.01% and 2% is covered by glaciers.

Rainwater Harvesting

Rainwater harvesting is the activity of direct collection or storage of rainwater into dugs, wells etc. Rainwater can be stored for direct use or can be recharged into the groundwater aquifer. It helps to overcome water scarcity.

Purposes of rainwater harvesting:

- To conserve and encourage the storage of groundwater
- To reduce water table depletion
- To improve the quality of groundwater
- To arrest sea water intrusion in coastal areas
- To avoid flood and water stagnation in urban areas
- To meet increasing demand of water.

Methods of Rainwater Harvesting

There are two important methods for rainwater harvesting:

1. ***Surface runoff harvesting:*** In urban areas, during rain surface water flows off. This water can be stored and conserved and can be used to recharge aquifers by using appropriate methods.

2. ***Rooftop rainwater harvesting:*** It is another method of conserving rainwater. In this method the rainwater is collected from roof of house/ building, surface of ground or pavement and stored in either a tank or diverted to artificial recharge system. This is less expensive, effective method to raise the groundwater level.

Components of Rooftop Rainwater Harvesting

- ***Catchment:*** The surface of roof of building, ground, courtyard etc. which receives rainfall directly is called catchment.
- ***Transportation:*** From the surface of catchment rainwater is carried to tank or storage area through pipes or slopes.
- ***First flush:*** The first shower of rain is flush off to avoid contaminating impurities of catchment surface present in rainwater. Provisions of first rain separator should be made at outlet of each drain pipe.
- ***Filter:*** The rainwater should pass through filter to effectively remove turbidity, color, microorganisms and impurities before storage.

  There are various types of filters available which are used to filter rainwater before harvesting.

  - ***Sand gravel filter (Fig. 3.1):*** This is common method of filtration where water is filtered by using pebbles, gravel and sand layers. Each layer of material is separated by wire mesh trough which rainwater passes before storage to separate impurities.

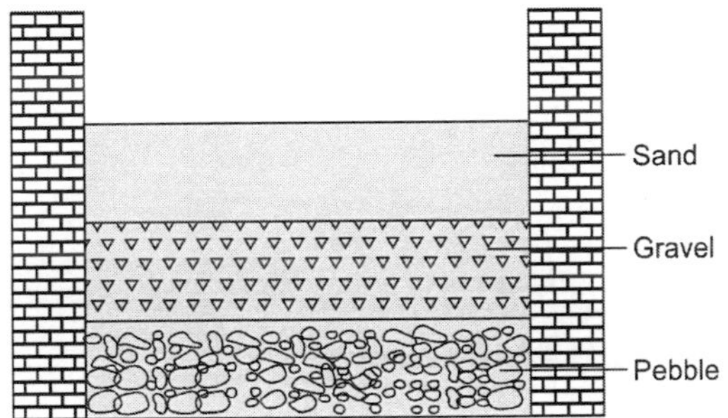

Fig. 3.1: Sand gravel filter

  - ***Charcoal filter (Fig. 3.2):*** Charcoal filter apparently work to sand gravel filter except by using another layer of charcoal in filter for cleaning and removing odor from rain water. This filter is also implanted in drums and each material layer is separated by wire mesh.

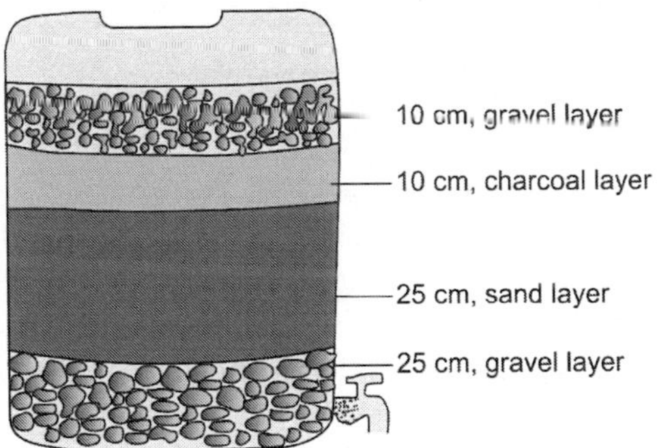

Fig. 3.2: Charcoal filter

- ***PVC pipe filter (Fig. 3.3):*** In this filtration method PVC pipe is used to filter rain water with inlet at one end and outlet at another end. Pipe is divided into three compartments by using wire mesh and each compartment is filled with sand, gravel and charcoal, respectively. Use of charcoal is optional in this filter.

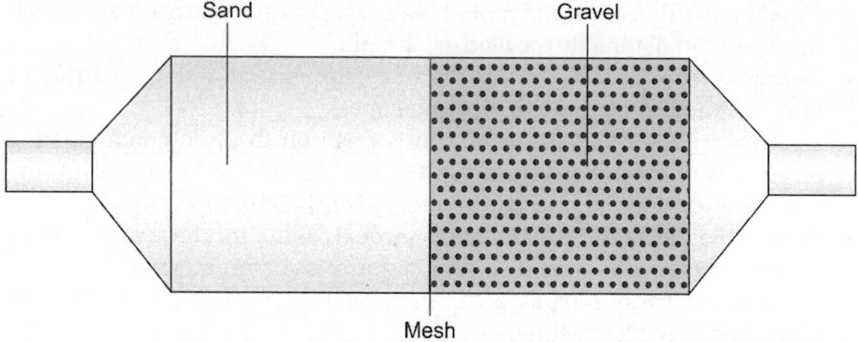

Fig. 3.3: PVC pipe filter

- ***Sponge filter (Fig. 3.4):*** This type of filtration is done by using PVC drum which have sponge in the middle of drum. This method of filtration is easy, less expensive and suitable for residential roof rainwater harvesting.

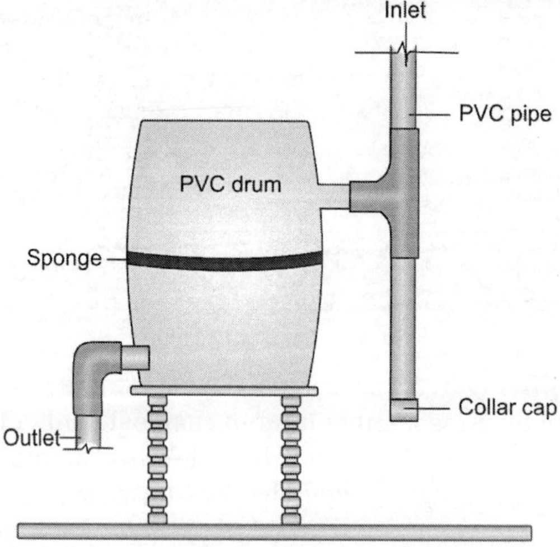

Fig. 3.4: Sponge filter

Types of Water

Water can be classified into two types:

1. ***Hard water:*** Hard water is enriched in minerals specifically in calcium and magnesium. If hard water is waste of industry become too dangerous. It has certain benefits because of enriched in minerals, it reduces solubility of potentially toxic metals such as lead, and copper. But it creates problem with use of detergent. It does not form leather when used with soap as well as leaves scales after wash.

Hard water can be changed into soft water after treatment including exchange of ions.

2. ***Soft water:*** Water contains little or no dissolving salts of calcium or magnesium is considered to be soft and safe water.

   Soft water is the water which is used for drinking because it contains sodium or minerals and have good taste. It has no dangerous effects on health and does not leave any scales or deposits after wash. It forms good leather with use of detergent.

Physical Characteristics of Water

- ***Turbidity of water:*** Turbidity is measurement of amount of transparency which water has lost due to presence of suspended particles. Turbidity of water is measured by using turbid meter and units for turbidity are NTU (Nephelometric turbidity units).
- ***Color of water:*** Water is a transparent liquid but it reflects blue color because of scattered light absorbed by water is returned to surface and gives appearance of blue. If color of water changes to dull and dark color then it could be dangerous for flora and fauna. The color of water is determined by using tintometer.
- ***Taste and odor of water:*** In general good quality water is tasteless and odorless. The extent of taste and odor measured in water sample is known as odor intensity and is related with threshold odor number. In public supplies water should be odor free and minimum odor no. is 1 which should not exceed 3 for good quality of water.
- ***Temperature:*** For public supplies temperature of water 10°C is desirable which should not exceed 25°C.
- ***Specific conductivity:*** Specific conductivity indicates amount of ions dissolved in water and can be measured as how well water conducts electrical current. The electrical conductivity of deionizer water is 5.5 μs/m and for drinking water range of conductivity should be 5–50 mS/m.

Chemical Characteristics of Water

- ***Total solids and suspended solids:*** Total solids (suspended solids + dissolved solids) can be measured by residue after evaporation of water from sample. The permissible amount of total solids in good quality water is 500 ppm.
- ***pH value of water:*** pH of water indicates presence of H^+ ions in water sample. The normal pH value of water is between 6.6 and 8.4 and pH of water is measured by using potentiometer.
- ***Hardness of water:*** Hardness of water is caused by presence of sulfates, chlorides, nitrites, calcium and magnesium present in water. For public supply the desirable hardness of water is 75–115 ppm.
- ***Chloride content:*** The chloride content of water can be measured by titrating the water with standard silver nitrate solution using potassium chromate as indicator. The chloride content of treated water to be supplied to the public should not exceed a value of about 250 ppm.
- ***Nitrogen content:*** Nitrogen in water can be present in any form like free ammonia, nitrites, nitrates and organic matter, etc. The presence of high

content of nitrogen in public supply can cause disease methemoglobinemia in infants. The desirable amount of nitrogen contents in public supply is 45 mg/ L.

Characteristics of Safe Drinking Water

The quality of drinking water can be measured by measuring following qualities of water:

- ***Contaminant free:*** The water is filtered of unhealthy toxins, including synthetic chemicals, toxic metals, bacteria and viruses, radioactive substances and other treatment additives such as chlorine and fluoride
- ***Mineral rich:*** The natural occurring minerals in the source water are not removed through purification processes, such as reverse osmosis and distillation.
- ***Alkaline pH:*** The drinking water has an alkaline pH between 7.0 and 9.5, which means that the water contains a healthy level of alkaline minerals such as calcium and magnesium.
- ***Micro-clustered:*** Water that is electrolyzed or 'reduced' will have smaller groupings of water molecules. Drinking reduced water can improve cellular hydration and cell-water turnover (i.e. nutrients into the cells and toxins out).
- ***Anti-oxidant:*** Water that is ionized has a negative oxidation reduction potential (-ORP) and thus acts to neutralize free radicals in the body and slows the oxidation (i.e. aging) process in the body.
- ***Good taste:*** The taste of water should be good to drink enough amount of water on regular basis to maintain normal health status.

Use of Water

Water is an important molecule for maintenance of life in biosphere. Water is a precious source of healthy life and for routine work. Humans, plants and animals are made up of mostly water.

Water is used for:

- For drinking purpose
- For household work like washing, bathing, cooking and cleaning etc.
- For building construction
- For the generation of steam for industrial use and electricity generation
- For the manufacture of hydrogen, oxygen and water gases
- For maintaninence of normal physiological processes of life
- For maintaninence of normal temperature in ecosystem
- For agriculture purposes
- For irrigation purposes
- For maintenance of aquatic life.

WATER POLLUTION

Water pollution refers to contamination of water sources natural and manmade which decreases quality of water and causes degradation of water for use. The contamination of water occurs when physical and chemical pollutants dissolved in water may be as a result of industrial waste or household waste.

Definition of Water Pollution

Water pollution can be defined as the addition of harmful chemicals and dissolvents in natural sources of water. This disturbs normal flora and fauna of water as well as put ill effects on health.

Or

A body of water, such as a lake, stream, river, pond, ocean and even the water underground in the soil, can become polluted when it is contaminated by sewage leaks, agricultural runoff or chemical spills and become unsafe for living organisms.

Sources of Water Pollution

Water pollution sources can be categorized into two parts:

1. ***Point sources:*** The point sources of water pollution are when pollutants leak from a discrete location like factory, sewage pipe and run off from single agriculture field which degraded quality of water in natural resources. The Bharat Petroleum oil spill in 2010 is an example of point source pollution, because the massive amount of oil leaked from a single point of origin.
2. ***Non-point sources:*** When water pollution occurs from addition of pollutants from various sources and contributes from a large area, e.g. one water source contaminated by multiple sources. The Mississippi river is at great risk for non-point source pollution because it is so large and is exposed to a variety of possible pollution sources. In Indian scenario The Ganga River is long and broad and is at great exposure for non-point pollution sources like industrial waste, residential waste, rain water ground surface waste, agriculture waste, etc.

Categories of Water Pollution

Surface Water Pollution

Surface water pollution is the pollution of water sources those are above the ground like rivers, lakes, streams, oceans etc. The pollution of these sources occurs when rain water runoff carrying pollutants of industrial waste, agriculture field chemicals, domestic waste etc.

Surface water can be classified into two categories:

1. ***Nutrient pollution:*** When pollution is caused by nutrients and fertilizers of agricultural field which leads to overproduction of algae on surface of water sources which inhibit the immersion of sunlight causes less production of oxygen by under water plants effects aerobic respiration of marine organisms leads to death of organisms under water.
2. ***Toxic chemical water pollution:*** When pollutants comes from waste of industries, agriculture pesticides, petroleum product wastes, car fluids etc which causes toxicity of natural water sources is called toxic chemical water pollution which effects aquatic life as well as life on earth.

Groundwater Pollution

When water which is present below layers of earth gets contaminated is called groundwater pollution. There are various sources given below which causes groundwater pollution:

- ***Storage tanks:*** When leakage of storage tanks of gasoline, oil, chemicals or other liquids occurs this mix with water present below the layers of earth and cause serious contamination of groundwater results in ill effects of health on and below ground life.
- ***Septic systems:*** If septic tanks collecting excreta and organic waste of houses, building and offices is not properly constructed or attached with city sewerage system it seeped out and mix with groundwater causes organic contamination of ground water i.e. causes increase in number of bacteria, viruses or other microorganisms in ground water.
- ***Landfills:*** These are the places to dump waste material in huge amount or where garbage is to be buried. If surface of landfill is not solid and having cracks then unwanted material and microorganisms will seep in groundwater through soil causes contamination of groundwater.
- ***Chemicals and road salts:*** Chemicals, fertilizers, pesticides and salts used in making road seeped in soil with rainwater causes contamination of groundwater.
- ***Atmospheric contaminants:*** Since groundwater is the part of hydrologic cycle, contaminants in other parts of the cycle, such as the atmosphere or bodies of surface water can eventually be transferred into our groundwater supplies.

■ WATER CONSERVATION AND WATER SOURCES PURIFICATION

Water Conservation

Water conservation is a term used to save most important and vital inorganic molecule, i.e. water, required saving life on planet. Water conservation includes all the policies, strategies and activities made to sustainably manage the natural resources of fresh water and to protect water environment to save and meet the demand of present and future.

Definition of Water Conservation

Water conservation refers to the preservation, control and development of water resources, both surface water and groundwater and to prevent pollution of natural water resources.

Methods of Water Conservation

Water conservation becomes the need of the day to save present and future life on planet. Various efforts have been taken by governments of countries to save or conserve water by building dams, reservoirs, digging wells and by initiating recycling and desalination (removing salts) of water.

The most important and favorable methods are to conserve rainwater and to increase groundwater level by using various methods in India:

- House in part of western Rajasthan is built in such a way that each has rooftop harvesting system and water is stored in tank and utilized for daily life activities.
- Nowadays it became mandatory in urban areas to leave little exposed earth during construction of houses, roads and pathways for soakage of water in ground which will help in increasing water table and will recharge the groundwater supply.
- Town planners and civic authority in many cities in India are introducing bylaws making rainwater harvesting compulsory in all new structures. No water or sewage connection would be given if a new building did not have provisions for rainwater harvesting.

Easy Steps to Conserve Water

- Turning the water off when brushing your teeth or washing your hair can save a lot of water.

  Purchase water-efficient products and appliances for your home. This includes dishwashers, sink systems, bathtubs and more.
- Plant your garden in the spring and you can save since water requirement levels are less during this season.
- Do not use water to defrost foods. Although many people do use this method it requires a lot of water consumption to do this.
- Check for leaks. This includes the toilet and the sinks in the home.
- Cut off the water supply to any areas in the home that you are not using.
- Do not throw away water that has been used for washing vegetables, rice or dals use it to water plants or to clean the floors, etc.
- Do not use unnecessary water flow for washing of vehicles instead prefer to dry cleaning of vehicles.
- Judicious use of water for agriculture and gardening.

WATERBORNE DISEASES

Waterborne diseases caused by consuming contaminated contain algae and pathogenic microorganisms. Outbreaks of waterborne diseases often occur after a severe precipitation event (rainfall, snowfall). Any disease that can spread through contaminated water. The contamination can involve bacterial, viral or protozoa organisms.

Definition: Waterborne diseases are caused by pathogenic microorganisms that most commonly are transmitted in contaminated fresh water. Infection commonly results during bathing, washing, drinking, in the preparation of food, or the consumption of food thus infected.

Risk Factors

- Droughts can cause increased concentrations of effluent pathogens, overwhelming water treatment plants and contaminating surface water. Older water treatment plants are particularly at risk.
- Changes in ocean and coastal ecosystems, including changes in pH, nutrient and contaminant runoff, salinity, and water security that can

cause degradation of fresh water, particularly in areas where much of the population uses untreated surface water for daily consumption and activities.
- Increased frequency of intense extreme weather events can cause flooding of water and sewage treatment facilities, increasing the risk of waterborne diseases.
- Indirectly, the lack of water can cause pressure on agricultural productivity, crop failure, malnutrition, starvation, population displacement, and resource conflict.
- Changes can occur in the distribution and concentrations of chemical contaminants in coastal and ocean waters through the release of contaminants previously locked in polar ice sheets, or in runoff from coastal and watershed development.

Types

- ***Waterborne diseases:*** Diseases where water act as passive vehicle for microorganisms to reach out in agent and causes infection.
- ***Water washed diseases:*** Disease which occur due to less availability of water, poor personal hygiene and infections occur due to improper waste disposal.
- ***Water-based diseases:*** Infections occur due to ingestion of water containing hazardous microorganisms.
- ***Water-related diseases:*** Infections transmitted by insects living close to water.

The diseases related to water supply and consumption of contaminated water.

Biological

Common biological diseases are:
- ***Diarrhea and dysentery:*** Diarrhea is a disease caused by consuming contaminated water and very common in under five years age children. This causes about 2 million deaths every year among children with age under five.
- ***Intestinal worms:*** Intestinal worm ingestion occurs due to poor sanitation and consuming contaminated water and food. This can lead to malnutrition anemia and retarded growth depending upon the severity of infection.
- ***Trachoma:*** Trachoma is infection of eye caused by bacterium *Chlamydia trachomatis* caused by poor sanitation and contaminated water use. Trachoma can cause trichiasis leads to irreversible blindness.
- ***Schistosomiasis:*** Schistosomiasis is chronic waterborne disease caused by worm schistosoma also known as bilharzias disease. This occurs due to infestation of fresh water containing cercariae of parasites released by snails. Schistosoma causes hypersensitivity and bladder infections.

Chemical

- Common chemical diseases caused by water are acute toxic effects and fluorosis which may cause methemoglobinemia in infants.

- Cancer widespread life threatening diseases outbreak occurs due to chemical pollution of water by industrial waste and agriculture pesticides mixing in groundwater.
- Chemical like mercury, cyanide, sulfuric acid, arsenic and methyl mercury used for mining are mix with water sources and cause water pollution results in various human health diseases as well as marine death.

Classification of waterborne diseases are given in Table 3.1.

Table 3.1: Classification of waterborne diseases as per infective agent

S. no.	*Infective agent*	*Disease*
1	Viral	Viral hepatitis A, hepatitis E, poliomyelitis, rotavirus diarrhea in infants
2	Bacterial	Typhoid and paratyphoid fever, bacillary dysentery, *E coli,* diarrhea, cholera
3	Protozoal	Amebiasis, Giardiasis
4	Helminthic	Roundworm, threadworm, hydatid disease
5	Leptospiral	Weil's disease
6	Snail (aquatic host)	Schistosomiasis
7	Cyclops (aquatic host)	Guinea worm, fish tape worm

WATER PURIFICATION

Water purification is the removal of contaminants and microorganisms from raw water to water quality and to make water safe for consumption for human beings. Substances that are removed during the process include parasites (such as *Giardia* or *Cryptosporidium*), bacteria, algae, viruses, fungi, minerals (including toxic metals such as lead, copper etc.), and man-made chemical pollutants.

Water purification can be done at small scale and large scale.

Small Scale Water Purification

1. Household purification of water
2. Disinfection of wells

Household Methods for Purification of Water

Boiling

- Easy and less expensive method of water purification at home.
- Water must be brought to 'rolling boil' for 5–10 minutes.
- Removes temporary hardness of water.
- It kills all microorganisms like bacteria, spores, cysts and ova present in raw water.
- Taste is altered with boiling but it is harmless.

Chemical Disinfection

Bleaching Powder (Chlorinated Lime)

- Bleaching powder ($CaOCl_2$) contains chlorine with pungent smell
- Chlorine is very effective against bacteria, viruses and fungi which are pathogenic for human health.

- Removes chemical compounds that have unpleasant tastes and hinder disinfection.
- Principle in chlorination is to remove a free residual chlorine of 0.5 mL/lit at the end of 1 hour of contact.

Chlorine Solution

- Chlorine is prepared from bleaching powder.
- Chlorine is applied on massive scale.
- Chlorine is very reactive element and forms compound with other elements of water.
- Chlorine levels up to 4 milligrams per liter are safe amount to mix in drinking water.

High Test Hypochlorite

- Hypochlorite is a calcium compound which contains 60–70% of chlorine.
- More stable compound than bleaching powder.
- 1 g of HTH with 70% strength is required to disinfect 1 liter of water.

Chlorine Tablets

- Chlorine tablets are extremely cheap method to purify household water.
- These tablets generate chlorine dioxide after coming in contact with water.
- 10 g chlorine tab generate 1 ppm of chlorine dioxide in 1000 L of water.
- It needs 4 hour treatment period for water before use.
- Chlorine tablets are used to purify drinking water in outdoor activities and emergency situations like disaster management sites.
- It changes after taste of water.

Iodine

- Available in the form of tablets.
- Can be used as an emergency disinfectant of water.
- When you are using iodine tablets you must be aware about water temperature.
- For purification of water within 30 minutes temperature of water should be 75°F and if need one hour then temperature should be 40°.
- Iodine effect persists longer than chlorine tablets.
- These tablets can be used only for persons with standard thyroid function.
- Each tablet contains tetraglycine hydroperiodide, which releases 8 ppm of titrable iodine.
- Two tablets treat one quart of water.
- Iodine tablets kill bacteria, viruses and giardia present in water.

Potassium Permanganate

- It is no longer recommended.
- It is a powerful oxidizing agent but not a satisfactory agent for disinfection of water.
- It may kill vibrio cholerae but not other types of bacteria.
- It alters the color, odor and taste of water.

Filtration of Water

- Filtration is an easy method used at small scale to purify water.
- Water filter which can be used are Pasteur Chamberland, Berkefeld filter and Katadyn filter.

- In Chamberland filters porcelain candles and in Berkefeld filters Infusorial earth candles are used for water purification.
- Ceramic filters are liable to logged with impurities and bacteria but does not kill viruses.
- Candles can be cleaned by scrubbing with hand under running tap water.
- Household water purifiers can be used working on method of reverse osmosis, e.g. kent, acquaguard, etc.
- This method is not suitable for water purification at widespread.

Purification of Water at Large Scale

At large scale water disinfection needs to disinfect raw water present at surface and ground of earth, e.g. wells, tanks, etc.

The following methods are used to purify water at large scale:

- Bleaching powder
- Double pot method
- Storage
- Filtration
- Disinfection

Bleaching Powder

- Bleaching powder is basically used to disinfect well's water.
- The required amount of bleaching powder can be calculated by calculating volume of water in well by using following formula:

  $$V = \frac{\pi D^2 h}{4}$$

  Where,
  V = Volume of water in the well (m^3)
  D = Diameter of the well (m)
  h = depth of water
  $\pi = 3.142$
- Roughly, 2.5 g of good quality bleaching powder is required to disinfect 1000L of water in well.
- Take 20 L of water from well in a bucket and add 300 g of calcium hypochlorite solution and keep bucket at rest for 20–30 minutes, when lime settle down pour solution without lime into another bucket.
- Now lower down bucket with chlorine solution vertically in well and after moving it below the surface of water violently mixes chlorine solution in well's water properly.
- One hour time period should be allowed before using water from well.

Double Pot Method

- Double pot method is used to disinfect well's water with chlorine in emergency condition.
- This method used two cylindrical pots with diameter 30 cm and 25 cm respectively and smaller pot is placed inside larger pot.
- A 1 cm hole is made in each pot, in smaller pot this hole is made at upper side near the rim whereas in outer pot it is made 4 cm above the bottom surface.

- A mixture of 1 kg of bleaching powder and 2 kg of coarse sand is prepared and slightly moistened with water. The inner pot is filled with mixture 3 cm below the hole and covered with polyethylene foil and two pots are lowered down 1 m below water surface. This mixture will work for 2–3 weeks and is advisable for 4,500 L water containing well.

Storage

- Storage of water is natural reservoir and considerable amount of purification takes place. The optimum time period for storage of water is 10–14 days.
- After 24 hours storage suspended impurities get settle down and water becomes clear which allows penetration of light into water and reduces microorganisms count.
- The aerobic bacteria present in water oxidize the organic matter by using dissolved oxygen and reduced free ammonia.
- The bacterial count reduced by 90% in water due to storage within 5–7 days.

Filtration

- By using porous media 98–99% of bacteria and other impurities can be filtered to purify water.
- Two types of filters are used: Slow sand or biological method and rapid sand filter.

Slow Sand or Biological Method of Filtration

This is a standardized method of purification used globally. The slow sand/ biological filter has following elements:

- ***Supernatant raw water:*** This method used sand bed as filter raw water through sedimentation, oxidation and particle agglomeration. The depth of sand bed 1–1.5 is used and downward flow of water through sand bed is allowed for purification. The process takes 3–4 hours time period.
- ***Bed of graded sand:*** Sand bed is most important part of slow sand filter with thickness 1 m and sand grains are used with diameter 0.2–0.3 mm. The sand should be free from clay and organic matter and supported by layer of graded gravel which is 30–40 cm deep and prevents water to carrying sand grains into drainage pipe. Sand bed provides vast surface area for filtration, i.e. 1 m^3 provides 15000 m^2 of surface area for filtration. The process takes more than 2 hours and filter water through sedimentation, absorption, oxidation and bacterial action.
- ***Under drainage system:*** Drainage system is present at the bottom of filter consists of porous and perforated pipes which serve the dual purpose of providing an outlet for the filtered water and supporting the filter medium above. Once the filter has been laid under drainage system cannot be seen.
- ***A system of filtered controlled valves:*** This part of filter comprised of various parts as below:
  - ***Filter box:*** It is an open box usually in rectangular shape, 2.5–4 m deep and built wholly or partly below the ground. The walls may be made up of stone brick or cement.

- ***Filter control:*** To maintain constant rate of filtration certain valves and devices are corporate in the outlet pipe system known as 'venturimeter' which measures the 'bed resistance' or 'loss of head'. When resistance build up operator opens the regulating valve to maintain steady rate of filtration and when loss of head exceeds 1.3 it is uneconomical to use filter.
- ***Filter cleaning:*** When bed resistance increases to such an extent that regulating valve is open up then it is time to clean the filter. At this stage supernatant water is drained off and sand bed is cleaned by scrapping the top layer up to depth 1–2 cm. After several years sand bed should be changed.

Rapid Sand Filter

Rapid sand filters available in two types:

1. The gravity type (Paterson type)
2. The pressure type (Candy's filter)

Steps of Process by Rapid Sand Filter

- ***Coagulation:*** Treated with a chemical coagulant like alum, dose varies from 5–40 mg or more per liter, depending on the turbidity, color, temperature and the pH value of water.
- Rapid mixing
  - Subjected to violent agitation in a mixing chamber for a few minutes.
  - This allows a quick and thorough dissemination of alum throughout the bulk of water.
- Flocculation
  - A slow and gentle stirring of treated water in a flocculation chamber for about 30 minutes.
  - Mechanical type of flocculator is most widely used.
  - It consists of a number of paddles which rotate at 2–4 rpm with the help of motor.
- Sedimentation
  - Led to sedimentation tanks
  - It is detained for periods of 2–6 hours when flocculent precipitate with impurities and bacteria settle down.
  - About 95% of flocculent precipitate needs to be removed before the water are admitted into rapid sand filters.
- Filter beds
  - Each unit of filter bed has a surface of about 80–90 m^2.
  - Sand is the filtering medium.
  - Effective size of the sand particles is between 0.4–0.7 mm.
  - The depth of the sand bed is usually about 1 meter (2–3 feet).
  - Below the sand bed is a layer of graded gravel, 30–40 cm deep.
  - The gravel supports the sand bed and permits the filtered water to move freely towards under drains.
  - The under drains at the bottom of the filter beds collected the filter water.
  - Rate of filtration is 5–15 m^3/m^2/hour.

- Filtration
  - As Filtration precedes the 'Alum- Floc' not removed by sedimentation is held back on the sand bed.
  - It forms a slimy layer comparable to the zoogleal layer in the slow sand filters.
  - It absorbs bacteria from the water and effects purification.
  - Oxidation of ammonia also takes place during the passage of water through filters.
  - As filtration proceeds, the suspended impurities and bacteria clog the filters.
  - The filters soon become dirty and begin to lose their efficiency.
  - When loss of head approaches 7–8 feet, filtration is stopped and the filters are subjected to a washing process known as back washing.
- Back washing
  - Rapid sand filters need frequent washing daily or weekly, depending upon the loss of head.
  - Washing is accomplished by reversing the flow of water through the sand bed back washing.
  - Back washing dislodges the impurities and cleans up the sand bed.

Programs and Legislation Related to Water Cleanliness

- In 1856, River Board Act was developed to control and for optimum use of water resources among interstate rivers.
- In 1954, Government of India launched 'Water Supply and Sanitation Programme' to provide adequate water supply and sanitation to whole country.
- In 1972, 'Rural water supply and sanitation' program was launched by government of India to provide adequate water supply and sanitation in rural areas.
- In 1974, Water Pollution Act for prevention and control of water pollution was passed by parliament.
- In 1981, Government of India launched international drinking water supply and sanitation program.
- 7th October, 2016, Indian government launched 'Namami Gange' project under name National Mission for Clean Ganga (NMCG).

AIR POLLUTION

Introduction of Air

Air is invisible but without it life would not be possible on earth. Air is the invisible gaseous substance surrounding the earth, mainly a mixture of oxygen and nitrogen. Air is earth's atmosphere which is making up of mixture of gases. The living organisms breathe in oxygen for respiration and breathe out carbon dioxide which is consumed by plants for photosynthesis. It has no color and smell but has mass and weight. Air creates atmospheric pressure.

Definition of Air

Air has mass and weight, invisible matter without odor and smell. Air is the invisible gaseous substance surrounding the earth, a mixture mainly of oxygen and nitrogen.

Properties of Normal Atmospheric Air

Physical Properties of Air

- Molecular weight of air is 28.96 lb/mol
- The specific gravity of air is 1.000
- Increase in temperature will change air/gas into vapors.

Chemical Composition of Air

- ***Standard dry air:*** Three gases nitrogen (78%), oxygen (21%) and argon (1%) form dry air. Standard dry air also contains a small amount of carbon dioxide, and very small amounts of neon, helium, krypton, hydrogen and xenon.
- ***Water vapor (humidity):*** The water vapor in air at ground level is almost 0–5%. The time and location also effects humidity level in air.
- ***Other constituents:*** The industrial, transformational and agricultural traces present in local air.
- ***Standard component of air:*** Carbon dioxide is standard component of air and amount of CO_2 in air depends upon location.
- ***Non-standard component:*** Non-standard components of air include methane, sulfur dioxide, nitrous oxide, nitrogen dioxide, ammonia.

Air Pollution and its Ill Effects on Health

The components of pollution present in air are not visible to naked eye. Air pollution is introduction of different particles specifically solid particles and gases into air of atmosphere which can cause health hazards. In urban area ozone is a major air pollutant when it mixes with air forms Smog.

Sources of Air Pollution

There are major four sources which contributes into air pollution as follows:

1. ***Automobile sources:*** The use of motor vehicles contributes into air pollution up to great extent. The common vehicles like cars, buses, plains, trucks and trains etc when they run on roads they emit hydrocarbons, carbon monoxide, lead, nitrogen oxides and particulate matter which converted into harmful oxidizing agents after coming into contact with sunlight. The levels of PM2.5 and PM10 (air-borne particles smaller than 2.5 micrometers in diameter and 10 micrometers in diameter) as well as concentration of dangerous carcinogenic substances such as sulfur dioxide (SO_2) and nitrogen dioxide (NO_2) have reached alarming proportions in most Indian cities, putting people at additional risk of respiratory diseases and other health problems.
2. ***Stationary sources:*** Stationary sources include the industrial air pollution sources such as power plants, oil refineries, factories and other industries emit carbon dioxide, ozone, hydrogen sulfide and sulfur dioxide which increases temperature of environment.

3. ***Domestic sources:*** Domestic sources includes various sources used in homes like burning of wood, coal, agriculture waste produces smoke, sulfur dioxide and nitrogen oxide. Households smoke pollution and to prevent government efforts.
4. ***Natural sources:*** Natural sources include windblown dust, wildfires and volcanoes etc. which contributes in air pollution.

Major Air Pollutants and Effects

The important and identified air pollutants are:

- ***Carbon monoxide:*** Carbon monoxide is produced with combustion of fossil fuels, cars, trucks, buses, small engines, wood which is poisonous in nature and decreases blood's oxygen carrying capacity causes slowing reflexes and drowsiness. Poison of carbon monoxide can cause headache, heart stress and death.
- ***Ground level ozone (O_3):*** The chemical reactions of volatile organic compounds (VOCs) and nitrous oxide in the presence of sunlight causes decrease in lung function and shortness of breath results in asthma.
- ***Lead:*** Metal refineries, waste burners and battery manufacturing industries damage fetal nervous system results in neural tube defects in children. It also causes cardiovascular and renal disorder in adults.
- ***Nitrogen dioxide (NO_2):*** The main effect of nitrogen dioxide is on breathing raised levels likelihood of respiratory problems. Fuel combustion worsens lung diseases and respiratory infection.
- ***Particulate matter (PM):*** Particulate matter is result of chemical reactions, fuel combustions, industrial processes; agriculture waste road construction waste causes heart and respiratory diseases.
- ***Sulfur dioxide (SO_2):*** High sulfur combustion, electrical and industrial processes and volcanoes produce sulphur dioxide aggravates asthma.

Control Measures of Air Pollution

The world needs innovative methods to reduce air pollution. Although, the atmosphere has several built in self cleaning processes such as dispersion, gravitational settling, flocculation, absorption, rain washout, etc. to clean the atmospheric air. We all take little efforts to make our air little cleaner such as:

- By using unleaded petrol. Prefer to use biodiesel or alternative containing less pollutants fuel and electric vehicles.
- Using fuels with low sulfur and ash contents.
- By using public transport, walk or using cycle, car pooling to prevent excessive use of vehicles contributes in air pollution. For example, the law of odd and even use of domestic vehicles in Delhi, implemented by Delhi Government to reduce air pollution due to transportation.
- Plant trees as they consume harmful gases from atmosphere and return oxygen, thus helps in making air clean.
- Industries and waste disposal sites should be situated away from residential area.
- Catalytic converters should be used to help control emissions of carbon monoxide and hydrocarbons.

- The use of high technology like Bharat -IV and Bharat-V to reduce emission air pollutants from transportation.
- The government of India has launched New Automobile Policy to prevent air pollution and to enhance preservation fossil fuels. As per this policy the government directed to manufacture low emission automobile and electrical vehicles. The new policy covered the duration of use of old vehicles (petrol and diesel) only up to 15 years.

Technical Methods to Control Air Pollution

Methods of Controlling Gaseous Pollutants

The harmful gases like hydrocarbons, sulfur dioxide, ammonia, and carbon monoxide can be controlled by using following methods:

- ***Combustion:*** This technique is applied when the pollutants are organic gases or vapors. The organic air pollutants are subjected to 'flame combustion or catalytic combustion' when they are converted to less harmful product carbon dioxide and a harmless product water.
- ***Absorption:*** In this method, the polluted air containing gaseous pollutants is passed through a scrubber containing a suitable liquid absorbent. The liquid absorbs the harmful gaseous pollutants present in air.
- ***Adsorption:*** In this method, the polluted air is passed through porous solid adsorbents kept in suitable containers. The gaseous pollutants are adsorbed at the surface of the porous solid and clean air passes through.

Methods of Controlling Particulate Emissions

The air pollution caused by particulate matter like dust, soot, ash etc, can be controlled by using fabric filters, wet scrubbers, electrostatic precipitators and certain mechanical devices.

- ***Mechanical devices:*** It works on the basis of following:
  - ***Gravity:*** In this process, the particulate settle down by the action of gravitational force and get removed.
  - ***Sudden change in the direction of air flow:*** It brings about separation of particles due to greater momentum.
- ***Fabric filters:*** The particulate matter is passed through a porous medium made of woven or filled fabrics.
  - The particulate present in the polluted air are filtered and gets collected in the fabric filters, while the gases are discharged.
  - The process of controlling air pollution by using fabric filters is called 'bag filtration'.
- ***Wet scrubbers:*** They are used to trap SO_2, NH_3 and metal fumes by passing the fumes through water.
- ***Electrostatic precipitators:*** When the polluted air containing particulate pollutants is passed through an electrostatic precipitator, it induces electric charge on the particles and then the aerosol particles get precipitated on the electrodes.

Some Other Methods of Controlling Air Pollution

- Tall chimneys should be installed in factories.
- Better designed equipment and smokeless fuels should be used in homes and industries.

- Renewable and non-polluting sources of energy like solar energy, wind energy, etc. should be used.
- Automobiles should be properly maintained and adhere to emission control standards.
- More trees should be planted along roadsides and houses.

AIRBORNE DISEASE

Life is dependent on basic elements water and air but natural and basic elements of life also convey death in certain circumstances. Airborne disease is one which transmitted through air. Airborne diseases are spread when droplets of pathogens are expelled into air through coughing, sneezing, or talking by infected person. These pathogens may be virus, bacteria or fungi. These pathogens enter through nose and throat and transmit infection through respiratory system. The spread of airborne infections depends upon three things: number of organisms, the virulence of organisms and the resistance of the individual.

Common Airborne Diseases

Common airborne diseases include following:

- **Influenza:** The seasonal 'flu' virus spreads easily from person to person. There are many strains of the flu, and it continually changes to adapt to the human immune system.
- **The common cold:** The condition called 'a cold' is usually caused by a rhinovirus. There are many rhinoviruses, and the strains change to make it easier to infect humans.
- ***Varicella Zoster:*** The common widespread disease like chickenpox caused by this virus spread easily through air from infected to healthy person. This disease causes small red spots on skin which turns into blisters and rashes within 48 hours after infection by virus.
- ***Mumps:*** Mumps is a contagious viral infection spread through air causes swelling of parotid gland and salivary gland.
- ***Measles:*** Measles or rubeola is a contagious viral infection occurs through transmission of infective viral from infected person after coughing and sneezing into air. This causes cough, fever, skin rashes, runny nose, red eyes and sore throat. Prevention is vaccination.
- ***Whooping cough (pertusis):*** Whooping cough is highly contagious bacterial disease transmit into air through cough of infected person.

Uncommon Airborne Diseases

- ***Anthrax:*** Anthrax is a bacterial disease caused by inhalation of anthrax spores. It causes nausea and flu symptoms.
- ***Diphtheria:*** A bacterial disease which damage the respiratory system and attacks on heart, kidneys and nerves.
- ***Meningitis:*** Meningitis is a viral infection, which causes inflammation of memranes of brain.

■ NOISE POLLUTION

Noise

Sound is normal feature for our life and is the means of communication and entertainment in almost all animals specifically in human life. The loud and disturbing noises those are without agreeable musical quality and sound creating irritation are factors behind noise pollution.

Definition of Noise Pollution

Noise pollution refers to term of such levels of noise or sound present in environment those creates irritation and disturbance to living beings.

Or

Noise can be defined as a loud sound that is unpleasant and unwanted. Noise is a physical form of pollution and indirectly effects to receiver, i.e. man.

Sources of Noise Pollution

Noise pollution has mainly two sources:

1. ***Industrial sources:*** The significant incline in number of industries resulted in creating noise pollution. The industries like textile mills, printing presses, engineering establishments and metal works etc. contributes heavily towards noise pollution. Industrial sources include the various noises those come from industries due to alarms, working heavy machines, overcrowding of workers, transportation, etc.
2. ***Nonindustrial sources:*** The nonindustrial sources include all other relevant sources than industries and factories those produce and incline environmental voices. These are as follows:
   - ***Transport vehicles:*** The automobile revolution brought various ailments for human life including noise pollution. Due to mushrooming in vehicles the traffic jams has increased resulting in excessive hooting of horns and voices of running engines impacted hugely to day-to-day human life.
   - ***Household:*** The indoor noises also cause internal pollution in homes that disturb, irritate and put ill effects among residents. The inside home noises like banging of doors, children's games, gadgets and crowding of people increase frequency of noises in home. Other equipment like mixer grinder, television, music systems, washing machines, air conditioners and refrigerators etc. aided the noises and produce noise pollution.
   - ***Public address system:*** The loud music systems those are used for an excuse of religious functions, celebrations, commercial advertisements etc. are excessively noise producing factors.
   - ***Agricultural machines:*** The various machines and vehicles used for agricultural purposes like tractors, thrashers, harvesters, tubewell motors, etc. significantly contribute in environmental noises to produce pollution.
   - ***Defense trainings:*** The trials for various defense equipment like guns, tanks, explosions, rockets also create noise pollution.

- ***Miscellaneous:*** The automobile repair shops, construction work, bulldozing, crowding of people, etc. are other contributors of noise pollution.

Effects of Noise Pollution

- ***Lack of concentration:*** The concentration needs conducive and peaceful environment for better output. But loud voices and irritating noises are stumbling block in high level concentration of workers, students and other people. Thus poor work output as well as continuous disturbance creates stress and diversion in attention resulting in poor results and ill efficiency.
- ***Fatigue:*** Because of continuous diversion of attention and poor concentration causes wastage of time and lack of continuity in work resulting in long working hours for completion of work that creates fatigue and health hazards among workers.
- ***Abortion:*** The pregnant lady always desire for cool, calm, safe and non threatened environment which is essential for growth and health of both fetus as well as mother. Noise causes frightened and irritable environment for pregnant lady sometimes result in spontaneous abortion and ill health among pregnant women.
- ***Ratings of blood pressure:*** Excessive and loud noises attack on person's peace of mind. Thus elevate stress level and increase pressure inside vessels causing hypertension that can result in fatal conditions.
- ***Temporary and permanent deafness:*** The effects of loud and unwanted noises result in huge effect on hearing sense of human beings. Mechanics, locomotive drivers, telephone operators, etc. all have their hearing, impairment as a result of noise at the work place. Physicist, physicians and psychologists are of the view that continued exposure to noise level above 80–100 db is unsafe and cause damage to occulomotor nerve resulting in temporary and permanent hearing damage.
- ***Effects on marine life:*** Because of use of ships, boats, oil drills etc. in oceans create excessive loud noises below the surface of water and disturb peaceful habitat and sensitivity of aquatic organisms that results in death of various species of fishes, whales and other organism.
- ***General health effects:*** Noise pollution causes anxiety, stress, headaches, irritability and nervousness among human beings.

Preventive Measures for Noise Pollution

Government's Role

- Laws should be imposed before giving authorization of license of various noise creating industries and factories to construct sound proof rooms and working halls to prevent access of voice outside the premises of industry.
- The use of excessive and unnecessary horns of automobiles should be banned specifically in residential areas.
- The noise producing industries, airports, bus terminals and railway stations should be constructed at outskirts of residential areas of cities and towns.

- Laws should be enforced to check excessive use of loud speakers during celebrations, religious functions and commercial advertisements to prevent inconvenience to public.
- Encourage and plan teaching programs for public regarding ill effects and prevention of noise pollution.

Community's Role

- People should gather information and awareness regarding noise creating procedures at home, ill effects and prevention of noise pollution in their homes and residential area.
- People should reduce use of automobiles by preferring pooling of cars, scooters, etc.
- During construction the sound proofs rooms for instillation of music system and home theatre should be preferred.
- Vegetation should be done inside and outside of houses, around the side of roads and in grounds because trees absorb noise.
- Early and timely service of automobiles and domestic equipment will help in reducing unnecessary noise during use of such equipment.
- Community folks should follow rules for silence zones like around hospitals, schools, colleges etc. by avoiding use of horns and loud music.
- Ban on use of firecrackers should be welcome to prevent pollution by all means.
- During construction of houses and buildings the control of noise should make to prevent inconvenience to other people.

SOIL POLLUTION

The soil pollution is a part of land degradation caused by presence of chemicals and other unnatural objects in soil's natural environment. The typical factors behind this pollution are agricultural chemicals or improper disposal of waste.

Definition of Soil Pollution

Soil pollution can be defined as the presence of toxic chemicals (pollutants and contaminants) in high concentrations into the soil that can pose a risk to human health.

Causes of Soil Pollution

Natural Pollutants

The natural processes that can lead to accumulation of toxic substances in soil which influenced soil quality as well as human health. The possible causes behind this may be complex soil environment, involving the presence of other chemicals and natural conditions which may interact with the released pollutants. Natural processes leading to soil pollution are:

- ***Natural accumulation:*** The concentration of certain compounds increased in soil due to imbalance between atmospheric deposition and leaking away with precipitated water, e.g. accumulation of per chlorate in soils in arid environment.

- ***Natural production:*** It occurs under certain environmental conditions like natural deposition of per chlorate in soil from precipitation of already present chlorine and metals with energy generated during thunderstorm.
- ***Leaks from sewer lines:*** The leakage of certain chemicals into subsurface from underground drain pipes of sewage mixes with soil, e.g. chloroform.

Man-made Pollutants

The man-made pollutants of soil are initiated by various processes like some industrial and some accidental. These man-made released pollutants into soil conjunct with natural process to form toxic soil. Certain man-made soil pollution processes are as follows:

- ***Accidental spills and leaks:*** During certain procedures like storage, transportation and use of chemicals they spill on the surface of earth mixes with soil, e.g. spilling of diesel at gas station.
- ***Foundry activities:*** During manufacturing of certain products those include use of furnaces resulting in possible dispersion of contaminants in environment and soil.
- ***Other human activities:*** Certain human activities like mining, agricultural, transportation and construction activities enhances mixing of unnatural chemicals into soil and increased concentration of toxins causes soil pollution.
- ***Chemical waste dumping:*** Illegal dumping of chemical waste into earth's surface increased chemical concentration of soil to highly toxic level.
- ***Landfills:*** During waste sanitary landfilling waste seepage down into the layers of earth and mix with soil as well as generate polluted vapors.

Types of Pollutants

The main pollutants of soil are biological and chemical.

- ***Biological pollutants:*** Biological pollutants include manures and digested sludge coming from human, birds and animal excreta.
- ***Agriculture pollutants:*** The soil is polluted with pesticides, fertilizers, herbicides, slurry, debris and manure coming from agricultural fields.
- ***Radioactive pollutants:*** Radioactive substances such as radium, thorium, uranium, nitrogen etc. can infiltrate the soil and create toxic effects.
- ***Urban waste:*** The domestic waste coming from garbage and rubbish material, dried sludge and sewage mix with soil causes pollution.
- ***Industrial waste:*** The waste of industries like steel, textiles, glass, cement, petroleum etc. increase toxicity level of soil in high concentrations as well as waste of paper mills, oil refineries, sugar factories, petroleum industries etc. causes soil pollution.

Control of Soil Pollution

- ***Control of soil erosion:*** Soil erosion should be prevented by increasing implantation of trees, because the roots of trees holds the soil and prevent floods and wastage of soil during rainy season.
- ***Proper hygienic conditions:*** Education programs should be implemented to regarding awareness of sanitary disposal in proper manner to prevent

mixing of toxins as well as rubbish in soil. For example, lavatories should be equipped with quick and effective disposal methods.

- ***Production of natural fertilizers:*** Biochemical pesticides should be used instead of chemical pesticides to reduce incline in toxicity of soil as well as organic agriculture method should be adopted. Awareness program should be organized for farmers about ill effects of chemical pesticides on health.
- ***Recycling and reuse of waste:*** The wastes such as paper, plastics, metals, glasses, organics, petroleum products and industrial effluents, etc. should be recycled and reused.
- ***Avoidance of packaging items:*** Government should make a policy to ban the use of plastic utensils and bags. Public should be aware about health hazards of plastic bags after discarding in soil and should be encouraged to avoid buying packaging material to prevent plastic bag waste.

MARINE POLLUTION

Marine pollution is a major problem of oceans which harm to life of aquatic as well as sea animals.

Definition of Marine Pollution

Marine pollution is caused by the entry of chemicals, particles, industrial, agricultural and residential waste into ocean and these articles have potential to increase toxicity level of sea water that can kill and cause life threatening hazardous to ocean animals.

Or

The introduction by man, directly, or indirectly, of substances or energy to the marine environment resulting in deleterious effects such as: hazards to human health, hindrance to marine activities, impairment of the quality of seawater for various uses and reduction of amenities.

Sources of Marine Pollution

The sources of marine pollution can be various type of waste comes from domestic waste, runoff surface water; agricultural fields, industries and sewage that mix with water in oceans and increased toxicity level of various particles as well as give birth to various aquatic toxins. The nuclear waste and electronic was dumped in ocean by governments of various countries that has created marine pollution by increasing toxin level of water in oceans resulting in deaths of various marine species.

Sources and Effects of Marine Pollution

Type	*Primary source/cause*	*Effect*
Nutrients	Runoff approximately 50% sewage, 50% from forestry, farming, and other land use. Also airborne nitrogen oxides from power plants, cars etc.	Feed algal blooms in coastal waters. Decomposing algae depletes water of oxygen, killing other marine life. Can spur algal blooms (red tides), releasing toxins that can kill fish and poison people.

Contd...

Contd...

Type	*Primary source/cause*	*Effect*
Sediments	Erosion from mining, forestry, farming, and other land-use; coastal dredging and mining	Cloud water; impede photosynthesis below surface waters. Clog gills of fish. Smother and bury coastal ecosystems. Carry toxins and excess nutrients
Pathogens	Sewage, livestock	Contaminate coastal swimming areas and seafood, spreading cholera, typhoid and other diseases
Alien species	Several thousand per day transported in ballast water; also spread through canals linking bodies of water and fishery enhancement projects	Outcompete native species and reduce biological diversity. Introduce new marine diseases. Associated with increased incidence of red tides and other algal blooms. Problem in major ports
Persistent toxins (PCBs, heavy metals, DDT etc.)	Industrial discharge; wastewater discharge from cities; pesticides from farms, forests, home use etc.; seepage from landfills	Poison or cause disease in coastal marine life, especially near major cities or industry. Contaminate seafood. Fat-soluble toxins that bio-accumulate in predators can cause disease and reproductive failure
Oil	46% from cars, heavy machinery, industry, other land-based sources; 32% from oil tanker operations and other shipping; 13% from accidents at sea; also offshore oil drilling and natural seepage	Low level contamination can kill larvae and cause disease in marine life. Oil slicks kill marine life, especially in coastal habitats. Tar balls from coagulated oil litter beaches and coastal habitat. Oil pollution is down 60% from 1981
Plastics	Fishing nets; cargo and cruise ships; beach litter; wastes from plastics industry and landfills	Discard fishing gear continues to catch fish. Other plastic debris entangles marine life or is mistaken for food. Plastics litter beaches and coasts and may persist for 200 to 400 years
Radioactive substances	Discarded nuclear submarine and military waste; atmospheric fallout; also industrial wastes	Hot spots of radioactivity. Can enter food chain and cause disease in marine life. Concentrate in top predators and shellfish, which are eaten by people
Thermal	Cooling water from power plants and industrial sites	Kill off corals and other temperature sensitive sedentary species. Displace other marine life
Noise	Supertankers, other large vessels and machinery	Can be heard thousands of kilometers away under water. May stress and disrupt marine life

Effects of Marine Pollution

- ***Oxygen depletion:*** Sea water is a huge source of oxygen, certain wastes like sewage and organic matter decomposition creates hypoxic conditions due to anaerobic respiration and deplete oxygen from sea water resulting in death of various marine lives, e.g. plants, fish and other aquatic animals.

- ***Choking marine life:*** The introduction of small plastic particles and bottles into sea water are swallowed by certain marine animals and these particles stuck in their throats causes choking as well as abdominal distention and halt digestive process results in death of fishes, turtles, etc.
- ***Higher acidity:*** Toxic chemicals make our oceans more acidic. Again, this makes them poisonous to marine life and causes harm to fish and marine mammals as well as marine plants and corals.
- ***Spoiling birds' feathers:*** The oil spilling in the water of ocean causes coating of oil on feathers of marine birds causes soggy feathers and due to that birds become unable to fly and feel difficult to float on surface of ocean resulting in deaths of various marine birds.
- ***Blocking out the sunlight:*** Pollutants such as oil or litter can block out the sunlight from sea plants which need sunlight for photosynthesis resulting in anaerobic respiration and increased level of toxicity.
- ***Dangers to human health:*** Human swimmers and water sports lovers can become endangered by swimming in a polluted sea. They can acquire various infectious disease of respiratory system and skin.

Control Measures of Marine Pollution

- Introduction of sewage treatment plants to reduce sewage sludge of final product before discharging into sea.
- Toxic pollutants from industries and sewage treatment plants should not be discharged in coastal waters.
- Cleaning oil from surface waters and contaminated beaches can be accelerated through the use of chemical dispersants which can be sprayed on the oil.
- Load on top system reduce oil pollution cleaned with high pressures jets of water.
- Crude oil washing: The cling age is removed by jets of crude oil while the cargo is being unloaded.
- Oil and grease from service stations should be processed for reuse. Oil ballast should not be dumped into sea.
- Spreading a high density powder over the oil spill, so that oil can be sunk to the bottom.
- Run off from non-point sources should be prevented to reach coastal areas.
- Sewer overflows should be prevented by having separate sewer and rain water pipes.
- Dumping of toxic, hazardous wastes and sewage sludge should be banned.
- Developmental activities on coastal areas should be minimized.

RADIOACTIVE POLLUTION

Radioactivity

Radioactivity is individual atomic essence and property exhibited by certain types of matter those release energy and subatomic particles spontaneously.

The release of any radioactive material into environment causes pollution and harms the biodiversity as well as human life. Radioactive pollution causes various cancers and mutations of DNA resulting in congenital health problems.

The India's single largest nuclear power plant is Kudankulam Nuclear Power Plant in a district of state Tamil Nadu. The construction of plant was started in 31st March, 2002 in collaboration with Russian state company and Nuclear Power Corporation of India and came into operation on 22nd October, 2013.

Definition of Radioactive Pollution

Radioactive pollution can be defined as the release of radioactive substances or high-energy particles into the air, water or earth as a result of human activity, either by accident or by design.

Or

Radioactive pollution can be defined as the release of radioactive substances or high-energy particles into the air, water, or earth as a result of human activity, either by accident or by design.

Sources of Radioactive Pollution

- Nuclear power plants
- Nuclear weapons and reactors
- Nuclear fuel cycle
- Radon gas emitted from earth's surface.

Causes of Radioactive Pollution

- ***Mining of radioactive ore:*** The process of crushing of radioactive ores like uranium, phosphate, etc. during process of mining releases radioactive waste and in high amounts is highly toxic.
- ***Decomposition of nuclear weapons:*** The process of decomposition of weapons containing nuclear material emits alpha particles as waste those causes radioactive pollution and high ingestion causes health hazards.
- ***Production of nuclear weapons:*** Radioactive materials used in this production have high health risks and release a small amount of pollution. The use of nuclear weapons in World War II has created huge damage in Hiroshima and Nagasaki.
- ***Coal ash:*** The coal known as dirty coal contain more radioactive substances. When this type of coal is burnt as fuel it releases radioactive waste in environment even the ash of this coal highly active in radioactivity emission and causes toxicity.
- ***Nuclear power plants:*** Nuclear power plants generally release low level of radioactivity in normal functioning due to safety precautions but during accident these plants release highly toxic and in large amount of radioactive substances in environment. The best example for this is the accident case of Chernobyl nuclear disaster in history and recent Fukushima, after the earthquake and tidal wave in Japan.

Effects of Radioactive Pollution

- Radiations may break chemical bonds, such as DNA in cells; this affects the genetic make-up and control mechanisms.

- Fatigue, nausea, vomiting and loss of hair (exposure at low doses of radiations, i.e. 100–250 rads).
- The bone marrow is affected, blood cells are reduced, decreased in body immunity, blood fails to clot, and the irradiated person soon dies of infection and bleeding (exposure at low doses, i.e. 400–500 rads).
- Higher irradiation doses (10,000 rads) cause damage to the tissues of heart, brain, etc.

Radioactive Waste Prevention and Management

There are four main techniques used for radioactive waste management:

1. ***Geological disposal:*** This is the process of dumping and burying of radioactive waste beneath the earth's surface for storage until it has decayed enough to not be dangerous any more. Previously radioactive waste was dumped into world's ocean but following the sixteenth meeting of London, Dumping convention of 1993, the dumping of radioactive waste into the sea is banned.
2. ***Transmutation:*** Transmutation of radioactive waste is the process of consuming the radioactive waste and turning it into less harmful waste. This process is not in regular use because of high cost.
3. ***Re-use of radioactive waste:*** The reuse of radioactive waste substances includes use of radioactive isotopes like strontium-90 and caesium-137 can be reused in food industries. This effort will reduce radioactive waste and is a ecofriendly management scheme.
4. ***Space disposal:*** This method is still not in use because of potential problems which can occur due to implementation of procedure. For example, a rocket used to launch the waste fails then huge amount of radioactive material will be released into the environment.

HOUSING AND VENTILATION

Housing

Shelter is everyone's basic need and this is met by making houses. The houses event us from climate change, dust, animals etc. The houses can be constructed in various types and with various materials e.g. wood, cement, bricks, sand and soil, etc.

Definition

House refers to houses or buildings collectively those known as accommodation of people where people used to live in.

Or

Houses are building for shelter and safety. These can be of different shapes, size and material.

Aims of Housing

- Shelter
- Access to community facilities
- Family life
- Economic stability
- Family participation in community life

Healthy Housing

- Housing provides physical protection and shelter would be healthy in nature.
- Provides adequately space and facilities for cooking, eating, washing and excretory functions.
- Provides for protection from hazards of exposure to noise and pollution.
- The healthy house's construction and maintenance will prevent from communicable diseases and promote health.
- Encourage community and personal development as well as strengthen personal and community relationships.
- The healthy house would be free from physical and psychological harm.
- The healthy house will prevent from ecological pollution.

Housing Standards

Social and Economic

- Social and economic characteristics such as family income, family size and composition, standard of living, lifestyle, stage in life cycle, education and cultural factors are taken into account.
- Because of cultural diversity and other factors such as climate and social traditions, standard of housing varies from country to country and from region to region.
- In short-there cannot be rigid, uniform standards.

Location and Site of Housing

- It should be elevated from its surroundings.
- It should have an independent access to a street of adequate width.
- It should be away from breeding places of mosquito and flies.
- It should be away from nuisances such as dust, ,smell, excessive noise and traffic.
- It should be in pleasant surrounding.
- Soil should be dry and safe for founding the structure and should be well drained.
- The sub-soil water should be below 1o feet.

Setback of House

- It is the open space all around the house which allows proper ventilation and lightening.
- In rural areas it is recommended that the built-up area should not exceed one third of total area and in urban areas it is allowed up to two-third of total area.
- At the back of house obstruction should not be there for lightening and ventilation.

Construction of Healthy House

- ***Floor:*** It should be pucca and satisfy the following criteria:
  - It should be impermeable, so that easy to clean and dry.
  - It must be smooth and free from cracks and crevices to prevent the breeding of insects and harbor age of dust.

    - It should be damp-proof
    - The height of the plinth should be 2–3 feet (0.6 to 1 mtr)
- ***Walls:*** The walls of house should be:
    - Reasonably strong, with low heat capacity and weather resistance.
    - Unsuitable for harbor of rats and vermin and not easily damaged.
    - Smooth (9 inch brick with wall plastered smooth and colored cream or white).
- ***Roof:*** It should not be less than 10 feet (3 mtr) in the absence of air-conditioning for comfort and with low heat transmission coefficient.
- ***Floor area:*** It should be at least 120 sq ft for more than one person and at least 100 sq ft for single person, floor area per person should not be less than 50 sq mtr.
- ***Rooms:*** It should not be less than two, at least one of them can be closed for security and the other may be open on one side if that side is a private courtyard.
- ***Cubic space:*** At least 500 c.ft per capita preferably 1000 c.ft.
- ***Windows:*** Every living room should be provided with at least 2 windows at height 3 feet (1 m) area should be 1/5th of the floor and one of them should open directly on to an open space
- ***Lighting:*** The daylight factor should exceed 1% over half the floor area.
- ***Kitchen:*** It must have a separate kitchen and should be protected from dust and smoke, provided with a sink for washing and proper drainage system should be there.
- ***Privacy:*** A sanitary privacy is a must for every house, belonging exclusively to it and readily accessible.
- ***Garbage and refuse:*** It should be removed from the dwelling at least daily and disposed of in a sanitary manner.
- ***Bathing and washing:*** House should have facility for bathing and washing belonging exclusively to it.
- ***Water supply:*** House should have a safe and adequate water supply available at all times.

Impacts of Poor Housing on Human Health

Poor housing is associated with the following health conditions:
- Respiratory infection
- Skin infection
- Rat infestation
- Arthropods
- Accidents
- Morbidity and mortality
- Psychological effects.

VENTILATION

Ventilation is replacement of vitiated air by a supply of fresh outdoor air which must be free from risk of infection and comprised of adequate humidity, purity and temperature.

Standards of Ventilation

- For proper fresh air supply the space should be from 300 to 3000 c. ft. per person.
- In a single room the recommended air change 3-4 times per hour that needs 100–1200 c. ft per person.
- The optimum floor space requirements per person must be from 50 to 100 sq.ft.

Types of Ventilation

Natural Ventilation

- ***The wind:*** The wind is an active force in ventilation. When it blows through a room, it is called perflation and when there is obstruction it bypasses and exerts a suction action at its tail end known as aspiration. The wind which blows from doors facing to windows is called ventilation.
- ***Diffusion:*** This is slow process of air passage through smallest openings.
- ***Inequality of temperature:*** Air flows from high density to low density and the higher temperature difference between inside and outside air increases the velocity of air.

Mechanical Ventilation

- ***Exhaust ventilation:*** Exhaust air is provided in large halls and auditorium. In this process exhaust fan creates vacuum inside room to extract fresh air from outside to inside and room air from inside to outside.
- ***Plenum ventilation:*** The air is received through ducts and desired points in air conditioned rooms. The centrifugal fans propel fresh air inside by creating positive pressure inside the room.
- ***Balanced ventilation:*** This is a combination of the exhaust and plenum systems of ventilation. The blowing fan must balance the exhaust fan.

Air Conditioning

- This is balanced air or the simultaneous control of air on humidity, air flow, bacteria, movement, distribution etc.
- Air conditioning is used in places where outside temperature is high than inside room.

ASSESSMENT

WATER POLLUTION

Essay Type Questions

1. Define water harvesting. Explain about various methods of water harvesting.
2. Describe about difference between hard and soft water.
3. Define water pollution. Describe in detail about sources of water pollution.
4. Describe about various methods of water purification.

Short Answer Type Questions

1. Discuss in brief about physical characteristics of water.
2. Discuss about various sources of water
3. Discuss in brief about various water borne diseases.

Multiple Choice Questions

1. The chemical formula of water is:
   (a) CO_2 (b) HCl
   (c) H_2O (d) H_2CO_3
2. Normal specific gravity of water is:
   (a) 1.0000 (4 °C) (b) 10.000 (4 °C)
   (c) 100.00 (4 °C) (d) None of the above
3. The units used to measure turbidity of water is:
   (a) SI (b) CM
   (c) KG (d) NTU
4. The desirable nitrogen contents in public supply water is:
   (a) 25 mg/L (b) 35 mg/ L
   (c) 45 mg/ L (d) 55 mg/ L
5. When water pollutants leak from a discrete location are called:
   (a) Point sources (b) Non point sources
   (c) Both (a) and (b) (d) None of the above
6. Schistosomiasis is caused by:
   (a) *Salmonella typhi* (b) *Clostridium tetani*
   (c) *Giardia* (d) *Schistosoma*
7. In infants acute toxic effects of Fluorosis causes:
   (a) Anemia (b) Meningioma
   (c) Methemoglobinemia (d) Thalasesomia
8. Chemical formula for bleaching powder is:
   (a) H_2Cl_2 (b) $CaCl_2$
   (c) $CaOCl_2$ (d) CH_2Cl_2
9. The amount of HTH (high test hypochlorite) require to disinfect 1L of water:
   (a) 1 g (b) 7 g
   (c) 4 g (d) 6 g
10. The objective of 'Namami Gange' project is to clean:
    (a) Ganga river (b) Narmada river
    (c) Gangotri river (d) Godawri river

AIR POLLUTION

Essay Type Question

1. Define air. Discuss about composition of atmospheric air.
2. Define air pollution. Describe about various sources of air pollution.
3. Explain various common airborne disease.

Multiple Choice Questions

1. The molecular weight of air is:
   (a) 28.96 lb/mol (b) 30.22 lb/mol
   (c) 25.15 lb/mol (d) 31.12 lb/mol
2. The industries and oil refineries causes air pollution, known as:
   (a) Automobile sources (b) Domestic sources
   (c) Stationary sources (d) Natural sources
3. The passage of particulate matter through a process medium of filled fabrics:
   (a) Gravity (b) Fabric filters
   (c) Wet scrubbers (d) Electrostatic precipitators
4. The solar energy and wind energy are:
   (a) Non-polluting sources (b) Polluting sources
   (c) Both (a) and (b) (d) None of the above
5. Diphtheria is caused by:
   (a) Virus (b) Fungi
   (c) Bacteria (d) Protozoa

NOISE POLLUTION

Essay Type Questions

1. Define noise pollution. Discuss in brief about various sources of noise pollution.
2. Describe in detail about harmful effects of noise pollution on human health.
3. Discuss in detail about various control measures of noise pollution.

SOIL POLLUTION

Short Answer Type Questions

1. Define soil pollution.
2. Enumerate causes of soil pollution.
3. Describe in brief about manmade soil pollution.

Multiple Choice Questions

1. The arid environment of soil occurs due to increased concentration of:
   (a) Per chlorate (b) Sulfur
   (c) Sodium (d) Fluoride
2. The soil toxicity increased due to radioactivity is known as:
   (a) Biological pollutant (b) Agricultural pollutant
   (c) Urban waste (d) Radioactive pollutant
3. The soil erosion can be controlled by:
   (a) Natural fertilizers (b) Plantation
   (c) Recycling of waste (d) Radioactive methods
4. Per chlorate is formed by precipitation of:
   (a) Sodium and chlorine (b) Phosphorus and metals
   (c) Chlorine and metals (d) Sulfur and chlorine

5. Soil pollution is a part of:
   (a) Land degradation
   (b) Water pollution
   (c) Soil erosion
   (d) Sanitary landfilling

MARINE POLLUTION

Short Answer Type Questions

1. Define marine pollution.
2. Enlist sources of marine pollution.
3. Describe in brief about control measures of marine pollution.

Multiple Choice Questions

1. Marine life includes animals live under surface of:
   (a) Water
   (b) Soil
   (c) Air
   (d) Sewage
2. The nutrient waste mixing in water enhances production of:
   (a) Fungi
   (b) Bacteria
   (c) Viruses
   (d) Algae
3. The coastal dredging and mining causes:
   (a) Cloudy water
   (b) Green water
   (c) Black water
   (d) None of the above
4. The persistent blossom of algae causes:
   (a) Nitrogen depletion
   (b) Oxygen depletion
   (c) Carbon depletion
   (d) Hydrogen depletion
5. The mixing and collection of oil on the surface of ocean block penetration of:
   (a) Air
   (b) Soil
   (c) Sunlight
   (d) Rain water

RADIOACTIVE POLLUTION

Essay Type Question

1. Define radioactivity and radioactivity pollution.
2. Discuss in brief about radioactive waste management.

Multiple Choice Questions

1. The India's single nuclear plant is situated in state of:
   (a) Punjab
   (b) Tamil Nadu
   (c) Maharashtra
   (d) Madhya Pradesh
2. The emission of high energy particles into air is known as:
   (a) Radioactive pollution
   (b) Air pollution
   (c) Noise pollution
   (d) None of the above
3. The process of mining releases the radioactive ore of:
   (a) Carbon
   (b) Hydrogen
   (c) Uranium
   (d) None of the above
4. The decomposition of radioactive weapons emits:
   (a) Beta particles
   (b) Alpha particles
   (c) Gamma particles
   (d) Theta particles
5. The recent nuclear disaster occur due to earthquake in Fukushima is place situated in country of:
   (a) India
   (b) United State
   (c) China
   (d) Japan

HOUSING AND VENTILATION

Essay Type Questions

1. Define housing. Describe in detail about construction of healthy house.
2. Define ventilation. Discuss in detail about types of ventilation.

Multiple Choice Questions

1. The building used as accommodation of people is known as:
   (a) House (b) Hotel
   (c) Office (d) Hostel
2. The house which is well ventilated, spacious and preserve from bacteria is called:
   (a) Ventilated house (b) Big house
   (c) Unhealthy house (d) Healthy house
3. At the location of house, the sub soil water should be below at:
   (a) 20 feet (b) 15 feet
   (c) 10 feet (d) 25 feet
4. The process of fresh outdoor air replacement with vitiated air is called:
   (a) Air conditioning (b) Ventilation
   (c) Diffusion (d) The wind
5. Exhaust ventilation is used in:
   (a) Small rooms (b) Closed rooms
   (c) Air conditioned rooms (d) Halls and auditoriums

ANSWERS

WATER POLLUTION

1. (c) 2. (a) 3. (d) 4. (c)
5. (a) 6. (d) 7. (d) 8. (c)
9. (a) 10. (a)

AIR POLLUTION

1. (a) 2. (c) 3. (b) 4. (a)
5. (c)

SOIL POLLUTION

1. (a) 2. (d) 3. (b) 4. (c)
5. (a)

MARINE POLLUTION

1. (a) 2. (d) 3. (a) 4. (b)
5. (c)

RADIOACTIVE POLLUTION

1. (b) 2. (a) 3. (c) 4. (b)

HOUSING AND VENTILATION

1. (a) 2. (d) 3. (c) 4. (b)
5. (b)

CHAPTER

4

Waste Management

Learning Objectives

At the end, students will be able to:
- Define waste.
- Describe the types of waste.
- Explain about various methods of solid waste management.
- Describe about biomedical waste and its management.
- Describe about waste water treatment.

WASTE

Definition

Waste is unwanted or unusable material which is discarded after primary use and is worthless and defective material. It may consist of unwanted material left over from processes of industry, commercial, mining, agriculture or domestic operations. The material may be discarded, accumulated, recycled or stored. It is refuse including garbage, excreta and sewage waste.

TYPES OF WASTE

Solid Waste

Solid waste is the garbage or refuse of homes or other places like papers, food waste, agriculture waste etc. Solid waste or garbage means all the waste which produces from cooking and consumption of food including animal and vegetable waste which can be decayed. The matter which is worthless and no longer wanted. Solid waste can be classified as follows:

Municipal Waste

Municipal waste includes household waste. This can further be categorized as:

Organic Waste

Organic waste contains municipal waste comprised of waste derived from household, industrial waste, commercial waste which is biodegradable. If organic waste is not treated properly or reused, it can cause serious threat to environment.

Types of Organic Waste

- ***Hydrocarbons:*** Things made up of hydrogen and carbon bonding and may be solid, liquid or gas in nature.
- ***Polychlorinated biphenyl:*** Waste made up of chlorine compounds, e.g. agricultural fertilizers in soils, hydraulic fluids, insulation fluids, transformers in paints etc.
- ***Insecticides:*** This is highly toxic organic waste effects through food chain, e.g. DDT.

- ***Detergents:*** This is highly dangerous domestic waste assimilated with ground water through sewage.

Chemical Waste

This sort of waste contains remains of old medicines, fertilizers, chemicals, sprays, polishes and batteries etc.

Recyclable Waste

This is conventional waste disposal which can be recycled into new useful material, e.g. papers, glass, metals, plastics etc.

Soiled Waste

This type of waste includes disposal of hospital like soiled dressings, clothes, gauges etc. with blood and body fluids.

Industrial Waste

Hazardous waste or disposal is specific in causing substantial or potential threat and danger to public health and environment.

The Environmental Protection Agency (EPA) has listed industrial waste into three types:

1. ***Non-specific source waste (F-list):*** It includes waste of common industrial and manufacturing processes, e.g. solvents which used for cleansing.
2. ***Specific source waste (K-list):*** Disposal or waste of specific industries like petroleum refining industries, pesticides manufacturing industries etc.
3. ***Commercial chemical products waste (P-list, U-list):*** When some unused form of chemical products like pesticides, medicines etc. are discarded causes hazardous effects in environment.

Biomedical Waste

Biomedical wastes are generally generated in hospital thus also known as hospital waste which may contain infectious material like infusion kits, soiled bandages, cotton, sharp instruments like needles, etc.

Definition: Any waste which is generated during the diagnosis, treatment or immunization of human beings or animals or in research activities pertaining thereto or in the production or testing of biomedical.

The types of biomedical waste are shown in Figure 4.1.

Objectives of Biomedical Waste Management

- To minimize the production/generation of infective waste.
- Recycle the waste after treating to the extent possible.

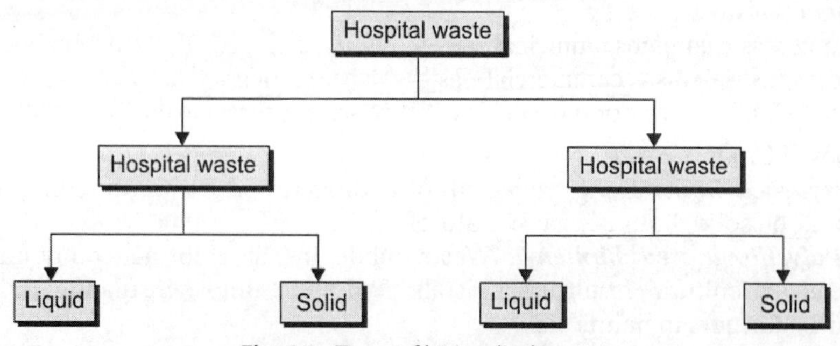

Fig. 4.1: Types of biomedical waste

- Treat the waste by safe and environment friendly/acceptable methods.
- Adequate care in handling to prevent health care associated infections.
- Safety precautions during handling the BMW.

Biomedical Waste Management (Fig. 4.2)

Incineration: The method use to dispose of dangerous and infectious hospital waste by burning. The waste is burnt at temperature 1300°C and burnt material is converting into heat, gas, steam and ash. The plant is known as incinerator. The steam generated during incineration is used for driving a turbine or generate electricity. The incineration reduces 20–25% of original waste and that can be used as clinker later on. A incinerator plant of 3000 tons per day capacity can generate 3 MW of power.

Management of Solid Waste

A solid waste management (SMW) system includes the generation of waste, storage, collection, transportation, processing and final disposal.

The components and waste material is categorized as following in solid waste management:

Municipal solid waste	***Materials***
Compostable	Food waste, landscape and tree trimmings
Recyclables	Paper, cardboard, plastics, glass, metals
Inerts	Stones and silt, bones and other organic material

The sustainable waste management hierarchy developed by earth engineering center at Columbia University which is widely used to sustainable solid waste management and disposal (Fig. 4.3).

Categories	Type of bag/ container used	Type of waste	Treatment/disposal options
Yellow	Non-chlorinated plastic bags Separate collection system leading to effluent treatment system	a) Human anatomical waste b) Animal anatomical waste c) Soiled waste d) Expired or discarded medicines e) Chemical waste f) Micro, Bio-technology and other clinical lab waste g) Chemical liquid waste	Incineration or plasma pyrolysis or deep burial
Red	Non-chlorinated plastic bags or containers	**Contaminated waste (recyclable)** tubing, bottles, intravenous tubes and sets, catheters, urine bags, syringes (without needles) and gloves	Auto/micro/hydro and then sent for recycling. Not be sent to landfill
White	(Translucent) Puncture, leak, tamper proof containers	**Waste sharps including metals**	Auto or dry heat sterilization followed by shredding or mutilation or encapsulation
Blue	Cardboard boxes with blue colored marking	**Glassware**	Disinfection or auto/ micro/hydro and then sent for recycling

Fig. 4.2: Rules for biomedical waste management 2016

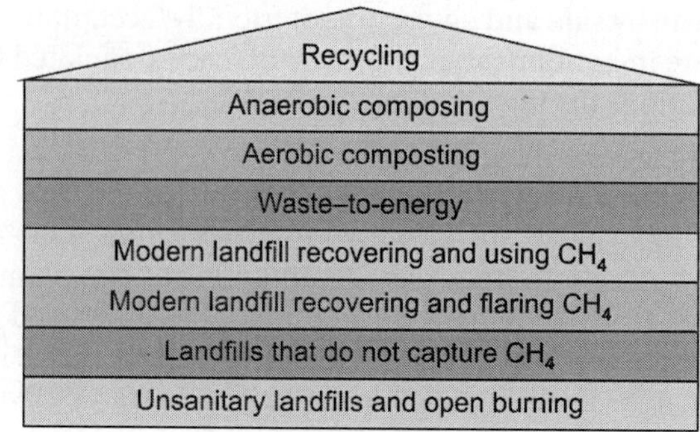

Fig. 4.3: Hierarchy of sustainable waste management

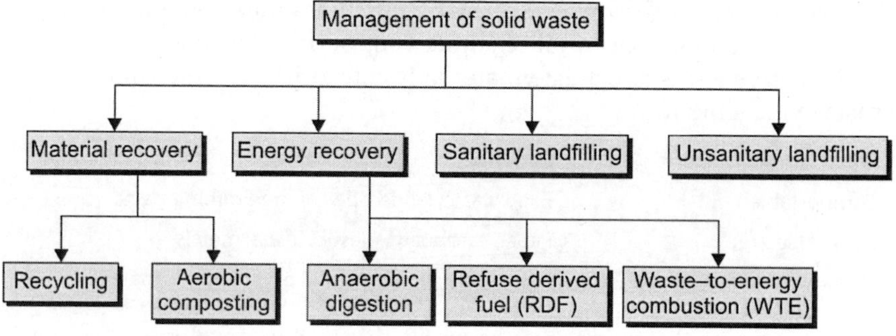

Fig. 4.4: Schematic diagram of solid waste management

Steps of Solid Waste Management (Fig. 4.4)

- Recovering of material
- Energy recovery
- Sanitary landfilling

Material Recovery

- ***Recycling:*** The reuse of waste material is an effective way to reduce solid waste. Recycling involves the chemical transformation of material. In this waste collected from household is used as raw-material to make new products (Fig. 4.5.).

Recycling of different material of waste

- ***Paper recycling:*** Paper waste includes books, news papers, magazines, cardboard and envelops are collected from homes, industries, market etc. and transported to industries for recycling.

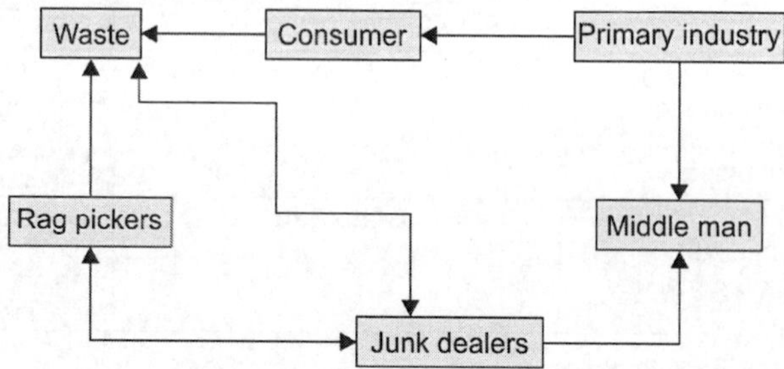

Fig. 4.5: : Recycling of material

Process of paper recycling

Repulping and screening
Paper waste is moved into vat (big paper grinding machine) and chopped small pieces are heated up after mixing it with water and chemicals to break and downing into fiber (organic plant material)

↓

Deinking
Fiber is washed with chemicals to remove ink and glue and this process is known as flotation

↓

Refining, bleaching and color stripping of paper is done

↓

Fiber is ready for new paper making

Glass material recycling

Collection of glass waste
(Collection is done from home waste, industrial waste, market etc. to drop at particular point)

↓

Cleaning and crushing of glass waste
(At processing plant, the contaminants like metal caps and plastic sleeves are removed and waste is crushed into small pieces called cullet

↓

Transportation of cullet to glass making factories

↓

In factories glass is mixed with soda ash, sand, limestone and heated at high temperature to melt it into liquid glass for making new glass

Aluminium recycling

Collection
During collection of waste from homes, market, industries etc. the aluminium waste is collected into different bin than recycling waste

↓

Preparation
At collection center a big magnet is rolled over the waste to separate steel waste

↓

Washing
After separation from other metals the aluminium waste is washed, crushed and condensed into briquettes

↓

Melting
The condensed aluminium is burn into furnace to melt for removing printing and designing known as Ingots

↓

Sheets
Ingots are fed into powerful rollers to flatten them into sheets for supply to can-making factories

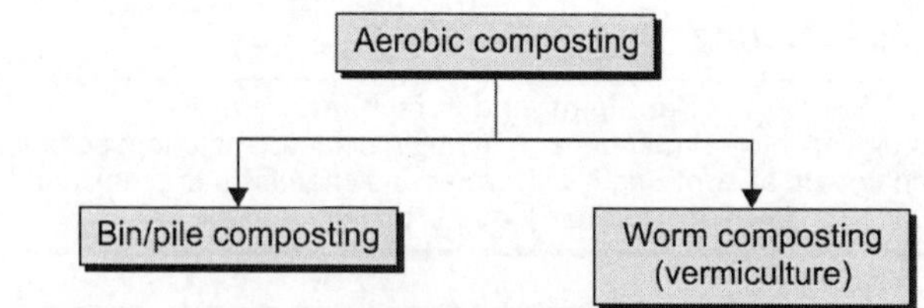

Fig. 4.6: Types of aerobic composting

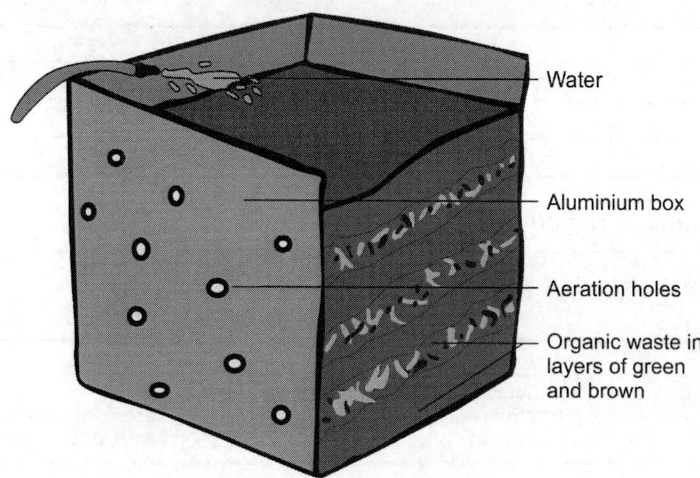

Fig. 4.7: Composting Bin/Pile

- ***Aerobic composting (Fig. 4.6):*** The organic waste like food, raw vegetables, livestock and poultry waste, sewage sludge are decomposed by bacteria, fungi, worms and other organisms, and this process is known as aerobic composting and decomposed matter is known as humus. The process can be categorized into two types (Fig. 4.6):
  1. ***Bin/pile composting (Fig. 4.7):***
     - Take an old bin or box and make holes around it for aeration
     - The organic waste must be cut down into small pieces
     - Separate brown waste (wood chips, sawdust, yard waste, dry leaves etc.) and green waste (grass trimming, fruit waste, vegetable waste, green leaves etc.) into different piles
     - Put waste into box, i.e. 50% brown with one upper pile and 50% green waste with lower at brown
     - Mix both types of waste with water after every 7 days
     - Wait for few weeks and compost will be ready for agricultural use.
  2. ***Worm composting (vermiculture)***
     - Take a bin and pick a spot to place bin where consistent temperature and moisture level is present. Avoid placing it near oven, heater or air-conditioner.
     - Drain holes in the bin for airflow.
     - Take two plastic blocks and place the bin on these blocks.

- Prepare worm habitat by preparing moist bedding. To prepare this take a newspaper or cardboard because these soak and retains moisture, this is necessary for survival of worms. Tear newspaper or cardboard into one inch wide strips and fill bin it with at least 8 inch high from bottom.
- Now soak worm bedding with water and make sure all the bedding is wet and then sprinkle dust on this bedding to provide natural habitat to worms.
- Put even layer of food and vegetable waste on top of worm bedding.
- Close the bin with lid for three days to two weeks to let the food decompose little bit before introducing worms in bin.
- When decomposition of food and vegetables started in bin leave the worms in the center of bin and close the lid.
- Add about ½ pounds of food daily in bin and wait for six months.
- When whole bedding is converted into compost then harvest it.

Energy Recovery

It includes recycle and reuse of municipal solid waste after treatment. Municipal solid waste always contains organic and inorganic matter from which fraction of energy can be recovered through various processes and treatment of waste. Various techniques used in energy recovery are:

- ***Anaerobic digestion:*** This is also known as bio-chemical conversion. It includes biogas and fossil fuel formation. During this process the microorganisms break down the organic waste like food scraps, manure and sewage sludge etc. in absence of oxygen and produce biogas. This biogas contains methane and CO_2, thus, can be used as fuel in kitchen or also can be converted into electricity by use of generator. The remaining liquid waste in plant can be used as fertilizer in agricultural fields.
- ***Refuse derived fuel (RDF):*** This is also known as thermochemical conversion and shred and burn. The waste which contains non-recyclable matter like plastic, paper, cardboard, labels etc. are used to produce fossil fuel.

  RDF is mainly used as substitute to coal in high energy industrial processes like power production, cement kilns, steel manufacturing etc.
- ***Waste to energy combustion (WTE):*** The process of combustion of solid waste to generate power like electricity, steam or other types of energy. The objective of this process is to reduce volume of solid waste up to 90%. This is the process of production of renewable energy technology.
- ***The residual*** as of combustion of waste used for making bricks and other construction material. This method has zero emission in the fly ash to save environment.

Sanitary Landfilling

Landfill is a rehabilitated land in which garbage and trash is buried. Sanitary landfill can be defined as the method of disposing of waste on land without creating hazards to public health or safety of environment.

Guidelines to selection of site for landfill: Sanitary landfill should always be away from:

- Highly porous soil.
- Steep slopes more than 20%.

- Source of surface and ground water.
- Three km away from airports
- 250 m away from commercial, residential and industrial developments.
- Areas with water, gas, electrical power and communication transmission infrastructures.

Unsanitary Landfilling

Unsanitary landfilling is characterized by open dumping of waste and this has lack of monitoring thus animals and birds feeding on the waste and has direct contact with environment.

It also communicates with groundwater by seepage through soil and mixing with surface water through aeration. All these factors cause pollution of environment and put ill effects on health of humans.

Water Waste Treatment

Waste water management is the field of treatment of water considered as waste from industry and domestic through recycling on to be disposed off in an environmentally conscious manner.

Definition

The process by any means mechanical or chemical used to modify the quality of waste water in order to make it more compatible or acceptable to human's use.

Or

The physical, chemical or biological processes used to remove pollutants from waste water before discharging it into a water body for reuse or discard.

Or

Waste water treatment is a process used to convert waste water which is water no longer needed or suitable for its most recent use into an effluent that can be either returned to the water cycle with minimal environmental issues or reused (Fig. 4.8).

There are two types of waste water treatment plants those can be used.

- ***Physical treatment plant:*** This plant operates on the basis of chemical reactions as well as physical processes to treat waste water. This treatment plant is used for water waste from industries, factories and manufacturing firms.
- ***Biological treatment plant:*** In the process of this plant the biological matter and bacteria is used to break down waste matter. Biological treatment plant is ideal for waste water from household and business premises.

Biological/Sewage Treatment Plant

Sewage is waste water from community containing solid and liquid excreta, derived from houses, street and yard washing, factories and industries.

Environmental effects of sewage water:

- It creates unpleasant odors and nuisance.
- Give platform to mosquitoes and flies for breeding
- This causes soil and water pollution
- It aided in incidence of diseases, e.g. enteric fever etc.

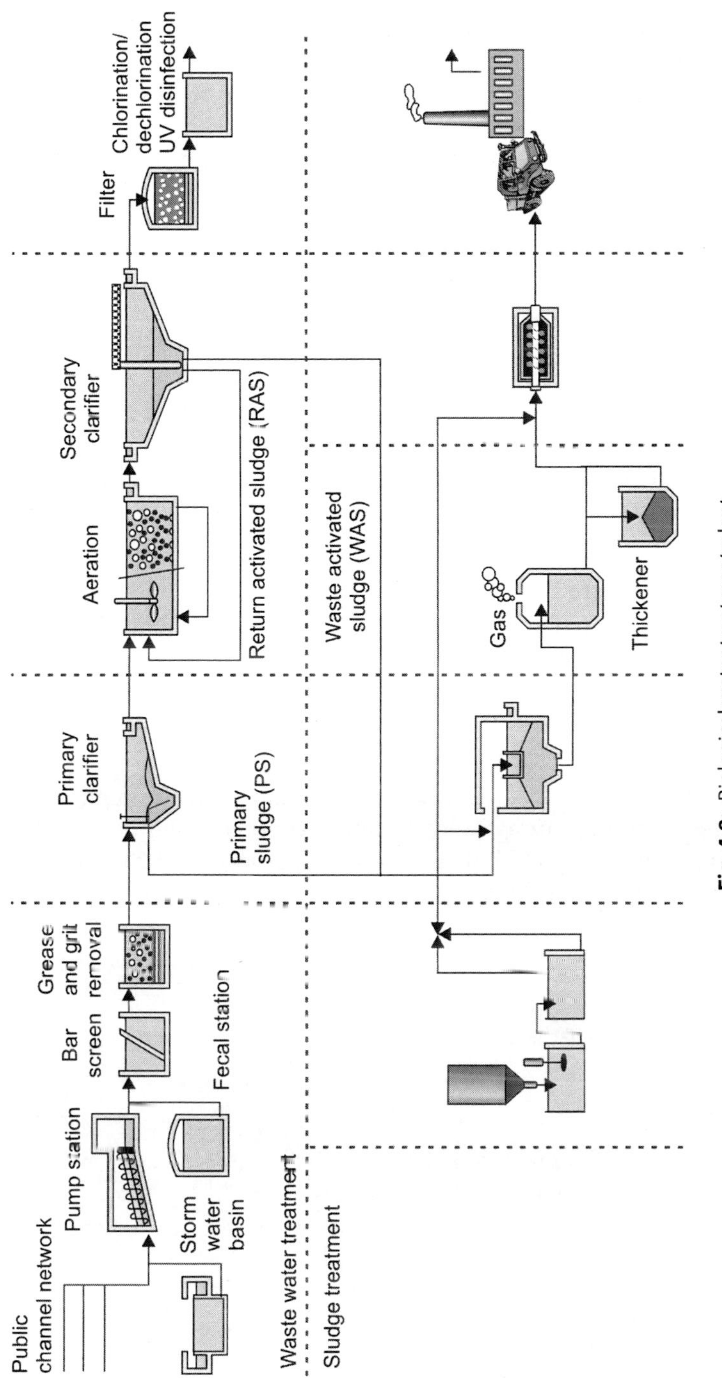

Fig. 4.8: Biological water treatment plant

Aims of sewage water treatment:

- To prevent mixing of sewage water into natural resources like rivers, sea etc. to prevent life of marine from toxic effects of sewage water.
- To stabilize organic matter to dispose of safely
- To improve quality of sewage water after treatment to dispose off in ecofriendly manner in rivers, sea etc.
- To remove suspended solids and organic matter from sewage water before reuse.
- To enhance decomposition of organic matter present in sewage waste water.

Decomposition of organic matter: The decomposition of organic waste in sewage treatment follows two processes:

- ***Aerobic process:*** The organic matter is broken down into simpler compounds like CO_2, ammonia, nitrites, nitrates and sulfates by action of bacterial organisms including fungi and protozoa with the help of continuous supply of dissolved oxygen.
- ***Anaerobic process:*** The present solid and concentrated particles are broken down into simpler form through decomposition with end products methane, ammonia, CO_2 and H_2.

Process of Sewage Waste Water Treatment

In modern sewage system, the water waste treatment completed in two processes (Fig. 4.9):

1. Primary treatment
2. Secondary treatment

Primary Treatment

- ***Screening:*** The waste water reached at treatment plant through drain pipes is firstly passing through metal screen where all solid objects like wood, plastics, sanitary pads, bottles, masses of garbage are removed from water to prevent clogging of treatment plant.

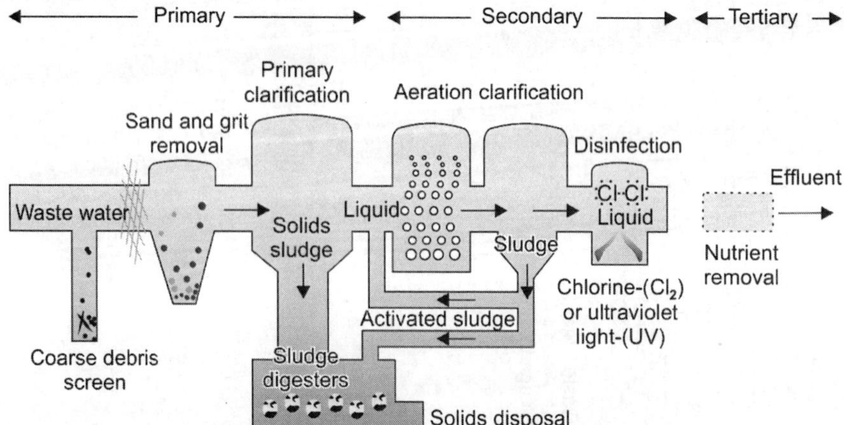

Fig. 4.9: Sewage waste water treatment plant

- ***Grit chamber:*** In next step the waste water pass through a 10–20 m long, narrow chamber with velocity of about 1 foot per second known as grit chamber or detritus chamber. In this chamber, the settlement of heavy solids like sand and gravel occurs for trenching and dumping.
- ***Primary sedimentation:*** In third step, the sewage collected into a huge rectangular tank for 6–8 hours where water flows at velocity of 1–2 feet/ min. Here sedimentation of suspended matter occur through which this result in
  - Settlement of solids at bottom due to gravity.
  - The organic matter (sludge) settles down and removed with mechanical devices.
  - During a biological process the present microorganisms in sewage breakdown complex compounds into simpler substances, e.g. ammonia, fat etc.
  - The fat and grease rise and collected at surface of water in tank called scum.
  - Then water is treated with chemicals like lime, aluminum, sufhate and ferrous sulfate.

Secondary Treatment

The sewage (effluent) from primary sedimentation still contains some organic matter and is highly anaerobic in nature.

This is further treated with aerobic oxidation with any one method among following:

Trickling filter method: A trickling filter is also known as bio-filter or biological filter. These are conventional biological waste water treatment units (Fig. 4.10).

Structure and function of trickling filter method:

The trickling filter is a cylindrical tank with high specific area filled with rocks gravel, shredded, PVC bottles and preformed plastic filter media and this high specific surface provide a large area for biofilm in which microorganisms grow and oxidize the organic matter of sewage into CO_2 and H_2O to generate new biomass. Next to this pretreated water is trickled over the filter with rotating sprinkle and cycles of water are being closed and exposed to air and oxygen is depleted in biomass.

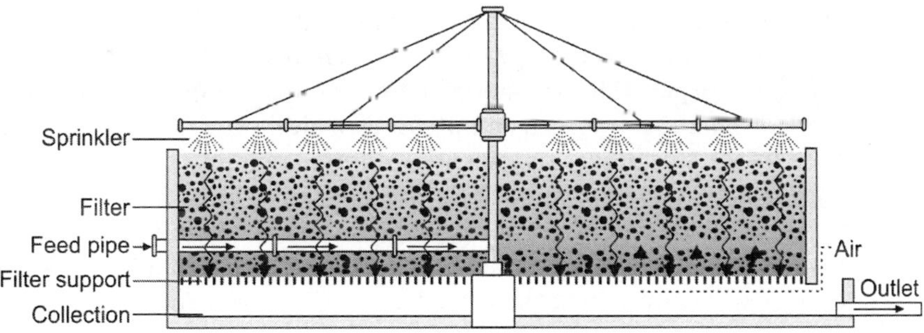

Fig. 4.10: Tricking filter method

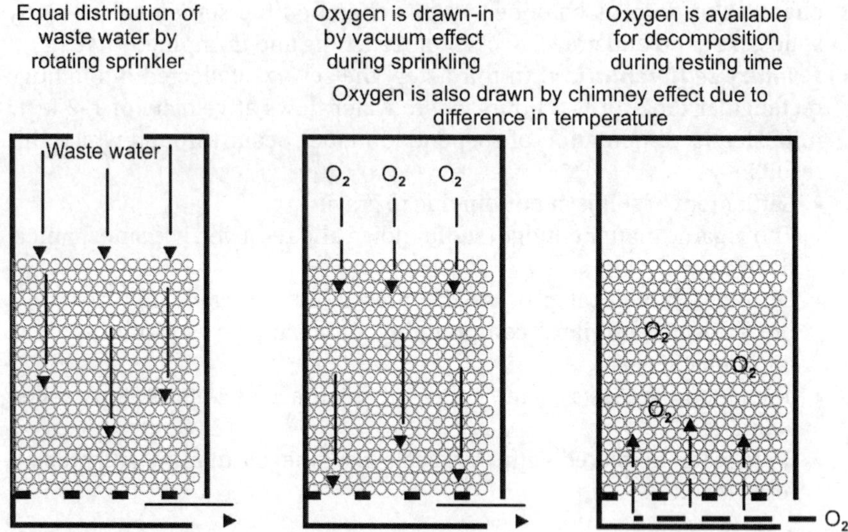

Fig. 4.11: Functioning of trickling filter

The filter is 2.5 m deep packed with tight plastic fillings. In this filter, oxygen is obtained through diffusion from air as well as from biofilm.

Principles of trickling filter: The trickling filter works on three principles (Fig. 4.11)

- Equal distribution of waste water by rotating sprinkles.
- Oxygen is drawn in by vacuum effect during sprinkle.
- Oxygen is available for decomposition during resting time.

Activated sludge process: Activated sludge process is a complex waste water treatment system. This term refers to suspended aerobic sludge consisting of flocs of active bacteria those consume and remove aerobically bio-degradable organic substances from screened or pre-settled waste water. This water treatment system is used for black water, brown water, grey water, focal sludge and industrial waste water (Fig. 4.12).

Procedure of activated sludge process:

- The effluent received from primary sedimentation tank is mixed with sludge drawn from final settling tank that is rich in aerobic bacteria.
- The mixture is expelled into aeration chamber for aeration through either mechanical agitation or forced compressing of air through bottom of tank or chamber and this process is known as 'diffuse aeration.'
- During aeration the aerobic bacteria oxidize sludge into CO_2, H_2O and nitrates.
- After aeration chamber sludge is led into secondary sedimentation tank for 2–3 hours. The aerated sludge is rich in bacteria, nitrogen and phosphorus that is good manure for agricultural field.

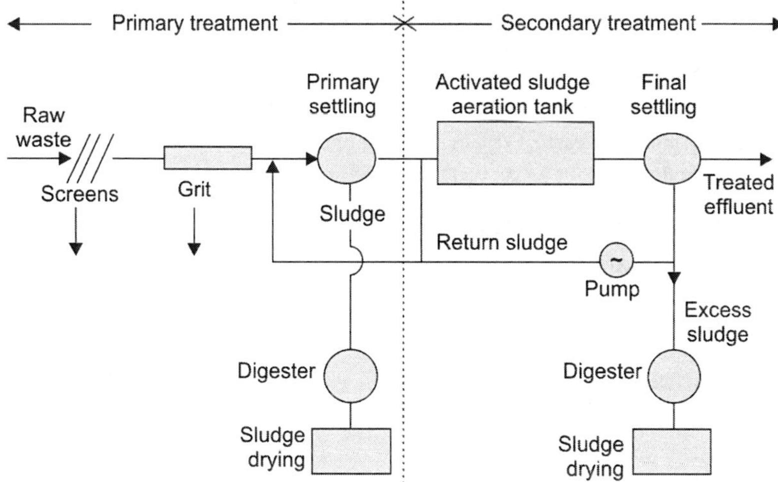

Fig. 4.12: Activated Sludge system

- The rest of sludge is subjected to sludge digestion tank for further treatment and disposal.
- In sludge digestion tank the offensive sludge is incubated for anaerobic auto digestion under favorable temperature and pH. After auto digestion sludge is broken down into CO_2, H_2O, methane and ammonia. The process takes 3–4 weeks and after making dry to sludge it became valuable fertilizer for agriculture and methane is used for heating and lightening purposes.

ASSESSMENT

Essay Type Questions

1. Define solid waste. Describe in detail about methods of solid waste management.
2. Define biomedical waste. Explain the rules of biomedical waste management.
3. Discuss in detail about waste water treatment process.

Short Answer Type Questions

1. Define waste water treatment.
2. Explain in brief about trickling filter method of sewage.
3. Explain in brief about paper recycling.

Multiple Choice Questions

1. The waste derived from household and industries is known as:
   (a) Organic waste (b) Inorganic waste
   (c) Biomedical waste (d) None of the above
2. The hospital waste is known as:
   (a) Organic waste (b) Inorganic waste
   (c) Biomedical waste (d) None of the above
3. Human anatomical waste is discarded in:
   (a) Red bin (b) Yellow bin
   (c) Green bin (d) Black bin
4. The reuse of waste material is known as:
   (a) Refused derived fuel (b) Waste to energy combustion
   (c) Recycling (d) None of the above
5. The removal of solid particles from sewage is known as:
   (a) Sedimentation (b) Filtration
   (c) Screening (d) None of the above

ANSWERS

1. a 2. c 3. b 4. c
5. c

CHAPTER

5

Ecosystem

Learning Objectives

At the end, students will be able to:
- Define ecosystem and concept of ecosystem.
- Enlist components of ecosystem.
- Describe structure and functions of ecosystem.
- Describe energy flow and material cycling within ecosystem.
- Understand the role of food web and food chain in ecosystem.
- Identify different types of ecosystem.

INTRODUCTION

Ecosystem is the community of living organisms, i.e. plants and animals who shares common environment. It is basically deals with the term ecology and environment.

ECOLOGY

The term ecology was coined by Ernst Haeckel. Ecology deals with studies of all lifespan on planet and their relationship with environment as well as with each other.

Levels of Ecology

- ***Biosphere:*** Biosphere is global ecological system integrating with all living beings and their relationships. It also studies interaction with lithosphere, hydrosphere and atmosphere. It includes total study of biodiversity on earth and processes like photosynthesis, respiration, decomposition, etc.
- ***Biome:*** Biome includes the study of large scale areas with similar flora and fauna as well as climate and containing communities with species that has adaptability to varying conditions in water, heat and soil.
- ***Biomes:*** The typical ecosystem spread over a large area containing some kind of abiotic (nonliving) and biotic (living) factors. Biomes can be classified as:
  - ***Terrestrial (land) biomes:*** Which can be further divided into desert, forest, grassland and tundra biomes.
  - ***Aquatic biomes:*** Which can be further divided into fresh water (lakes and ponds) and marine (oceans) biomes.

ECOSYSTEM

Ecosystem is the study of ecology. Ecology include only the study of living organisms only in biological means and relation with each other and environment while ecosystem includes study of whole environment of living organisms, their relation with environment and with each other by all means biological, physical and chemical (Fig. 5.1).

Definition

Ecosystem is the study of set of organisms and nonliving components connected by exchange of matter and energy.

Or

It is an integrated unit consisting of interacting plants, animals and micro-organisms whose survival depends upon the maintaninence and regulation of their biotic and abiotic structures and functions.

Or

Ecosystem is a complex in which habitat, plants and animals are considered as one interacting unit, the materials and energy of one passing in and out of the others. *Woodbury*

Concept of Ecosystem

Ecosystem = Biotic + Abiotic

The ecosystem is a unit or system comprised of a number of subunits which all are directly and indirectly linked with each other. The subunits of ecosystem are:

- ***Geographical ecosystem:*** The nature of ecosystem is based on geographical features such as hills, mountains, plains, lakes, rivers, islands etc. It also includes climatic conditions like temperature, pressure, rainfall, amount of sunlight, etc.

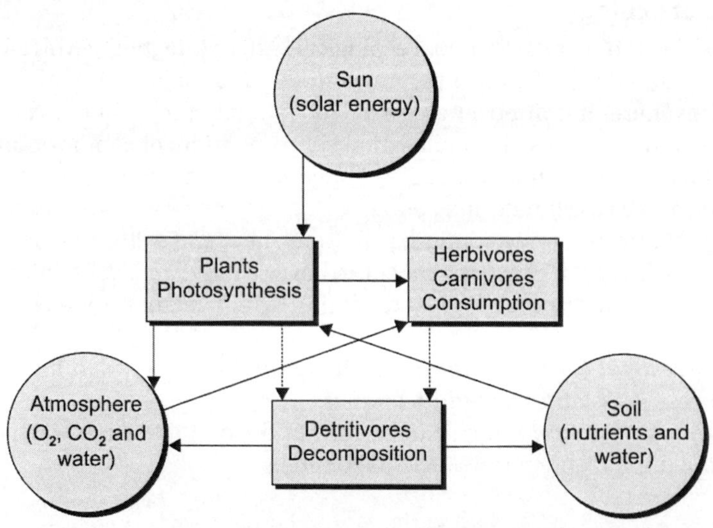

Fig. 5.1: Relationship within an ecosystem

- ***Community ecosystem:*** The study of interaction between species and abiotic environment and within species. It includes the study of effects of community structure and species richness, diversity and pattern of abundance.
- ***Population:*** It consists of groups of organisms from same species who interact and interbreed among themselves.
- ***Organisms:*** The smallest unit of study in ecology and refers to an individual member of a species, e.g. human.

Components of Ecosystem

Ecosystem has two major components (Fig. 5.2 and Table 5.1):

1. ***Biotic components:*** These are living components like plants and animals those interact with each other and environment.
2. ***Abiotic components:*** These are nonliving components of environments those interact with living organisms like temperature, sunlight, etc.

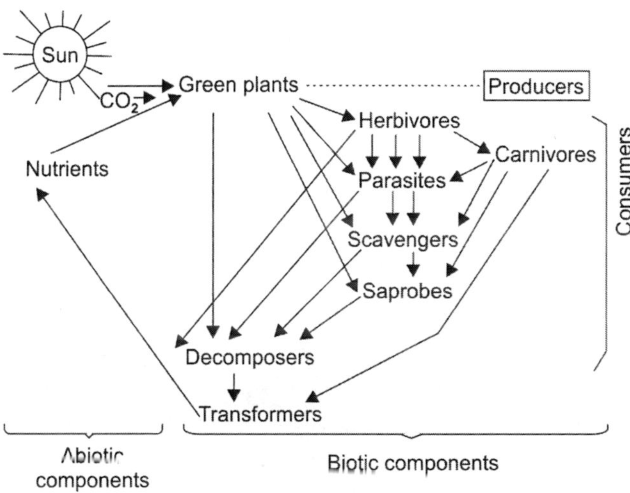

Fig. 5.2: Different components of ecosystem

Table 5.1: Difference between abiotic components and biotic components

Abiotic components	*Biotic components*
Nonliving components of environment	Living components or organisms
Includes inorganic substances like CO_2, H_2O, etc.	Includes organic components like plants and animals
Includes climatic factors like temperature, sunlight, etc.	Interact with climatic factors and take services from climatic factors in living processes like photosynthesis
These can be classified as inorganic material and climatic factors	These can be classified as producers, consumers and decomposers

Biotic Components of Ecosystem (Fig. 5.3)

- ***Producers (autotrophs)***
  - First trophic level components those make/produce organic energy resources from inorganic/abiotic components of environment, e.g. sugar formation through photosynthesis.
  - The plant produces an organic mass called **biomass**.
  - The primary production of biomass in ecosystem by producers comprised of two processes:
    i. ***Photosynthesis:*** The main producers are plants those converts energy from sunlight along with CO_2 and H_2O to produce sugar (glucose) and O_2.
    ii. ***Chemosynthesis:*** This is the method to produce energy from chemicals instead of using solar energy.
- ***Consumers (heterotrophs):*** The organisms at second trophic level those collect energy from environment produced by producers, e.g. oxygen and consume to perform respiration to give inorganic CO_2 to producers. These can be classified into three parts:
  1. ***Primary consumers (herbivores):*** The organisms who consumes producers (plants) as food, e.g. cows, buffaloes, etc.
  2. ***Secondary consumers (carnivores):*** The organisms those prey on primary consumers or other animals, e.g. lion, tiger, etc.
  3. ***Tertiary consumers:*** The organisms those consume secondary consumers, e.g. bacteria, etc.
- ***Omnivores:*** The organisms those consumes both producers and consumers for food, e.g. humans.

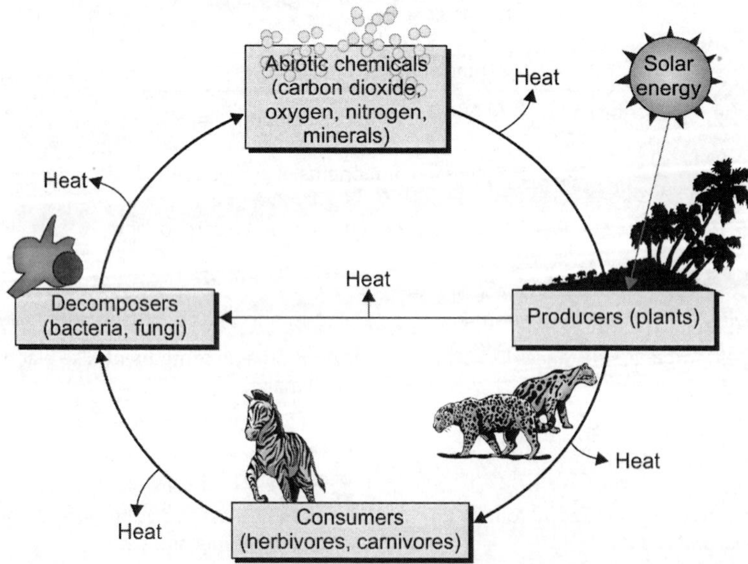

Fig. 5.3: Biotic components of ecosystem

- ***Deritivores/decomposers/scavengers:*** The organisms those consume dead tissues and organic waste, e.g. bacteria, fungi, etc.

Process of Ecosystem

The major fundamental prerequisite for life on earth is continuous flow of energy to keep biochemical process going on.

It is a fact that any kind of process will either require energy or release energy. On the earth major source of energy flow is the sun. Thus process of ecosystem or energy flow is based on thermodynamics. The basic principles or laws of thermodynamics are:

- The first law of thermodynamics states that energy may be transformed from one type into another, but it is neither created nor destroyed.
- The second law states that no energy transformations are 100% efficient, i.e. energy is always being transformed from more useful to less useful form.
- Under natural conditions, energy tends to flow from higher level to the lower level.

Energy in Ecological System

- The ultimate source of energy in ecological system is the sun.
- When solar energy strikes to surface of earth, it is converted into heat energy.
- About 10% of solar energy is absorbed by plants to produce food.
- This food energy flows through a series of organisms as food web and food chains.
- This energy flow process maintains ecological function.

Structure of Ecosystem (Fig. 5.4)

Ecosystem is self-sustained, functional unit. Ecosystem has following main structural features:

- ***Species composition:*** It includes differences between types of ecosystems based upon geography, topography and climate. Maximum species composition occurs in tropical rain forests and coral reefs whereas minimum occurs in deserts and arctic regions.
- ***Stratification structure:*** The composition of vertical layers (population) based on density of vegetation, e.g. deserts have vertical layers.
- ***Trophic structure:*** Each ecosystem has specific food chains and food webs.
- ***Standing state:*** The amount of inorganic nutrients present in water and soil at anytime in ecosystem.
- ***Standing crop:*** The amount of live biomass present in ecosystem.

Functions of Ecosystem

The ecosystem is a discrete, structural, functional and life-sustaining environmental system with abiotic and biotic components.

The basic process of ecosystem includes the production and exchange of energy. Thus ecosystem has following major functional components:

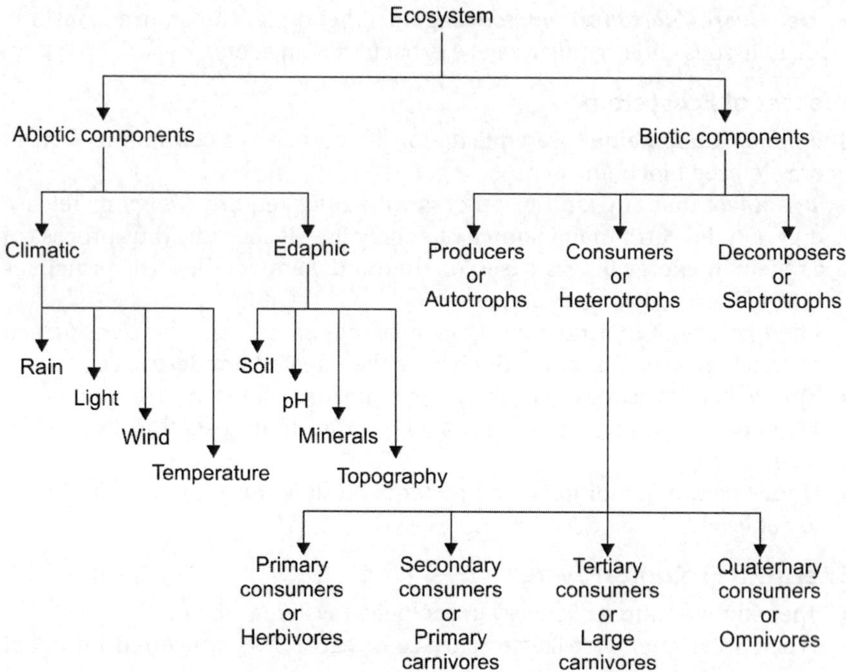

Fig. 5.4: Structure of ecosystem

- Inorganic constituents (air, water and mineral salts)
- Organisms (plants, animals and microbes)
- Energy input which enters from outside (sun).

Thus ecosystem has following principal operations:

- Reception of radiant energy of sun.
- Manufacture of organic materials from inorganic components by producers.
- Consumption of producers by consumers and further elaboration of consumed material.
- The decomposition of complex organic compounds by decomposers and convert these compounds into suitable forms for reutilization by producers.
- Maintenance of biological diversity and stability.

The ecosystem also has following major functions:

Trophic level interaction: Maintenance of ecosystem member's connections with each other by maintaining nutrient needs, e.g. food chain and food web.

- ***Food web (Fig. 5.5):***
  - This comprises of network of food chains as well as relationships of feeding by which energy is flowed or passed on from one species of living organisms to another called food web.
  - Food web represents description of relationships of feeding among species in ecological community, e.g. who feeds on whom.

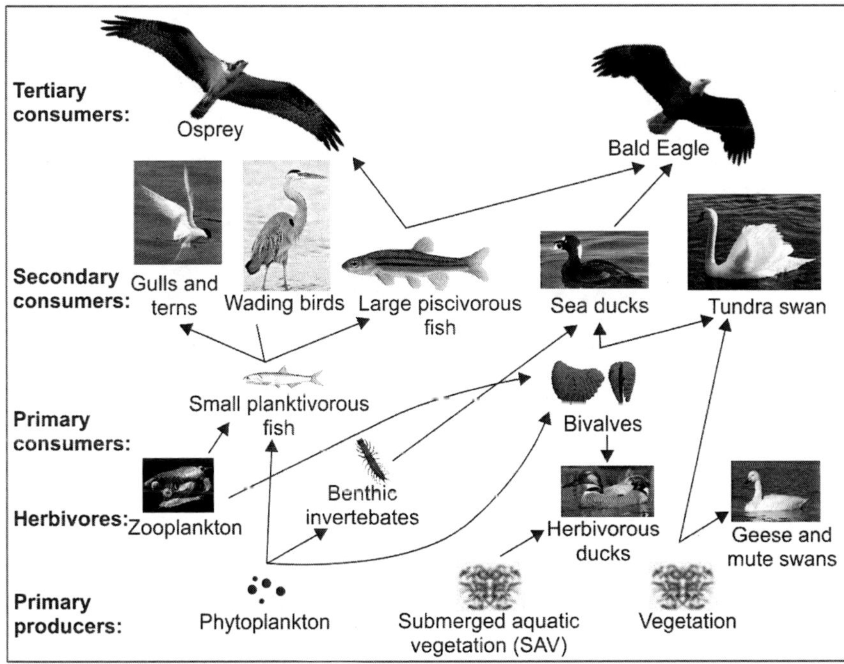

Fig. 5.5: Graphic representation of a generalized food web for some waterbirds in the Chesapeake Bay

- ***Food chain:*** Then sequential or systematic chain of eating and being eaten is called food chain (Fig. 5.6 and Fig. 5.7).
  Some organisms produce energy while others obtain it through feeding and decomposition that is known as food chain.
  - ***Ecological succession:*** It deals with changes in features and numbers of ecosystem members with time.
  - ***Biogeochemistry:*** It deals with maintenance of cycling of essential materials within ecosystem.

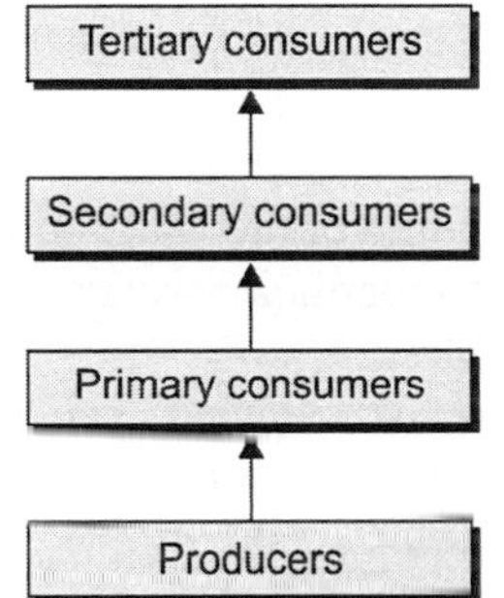

Fig. 5.6: Trophic level food chain

Energy Flow and Material Cycling in Ecosystem

In ecosystem there is a constant flow of energy between organisms. In cyclic manner material and energy is transformed from one organism to another in ecosystem.

There are specific cycles of energy flow that effect life of organisms in a particular ecosystem. These cycles are as follows:

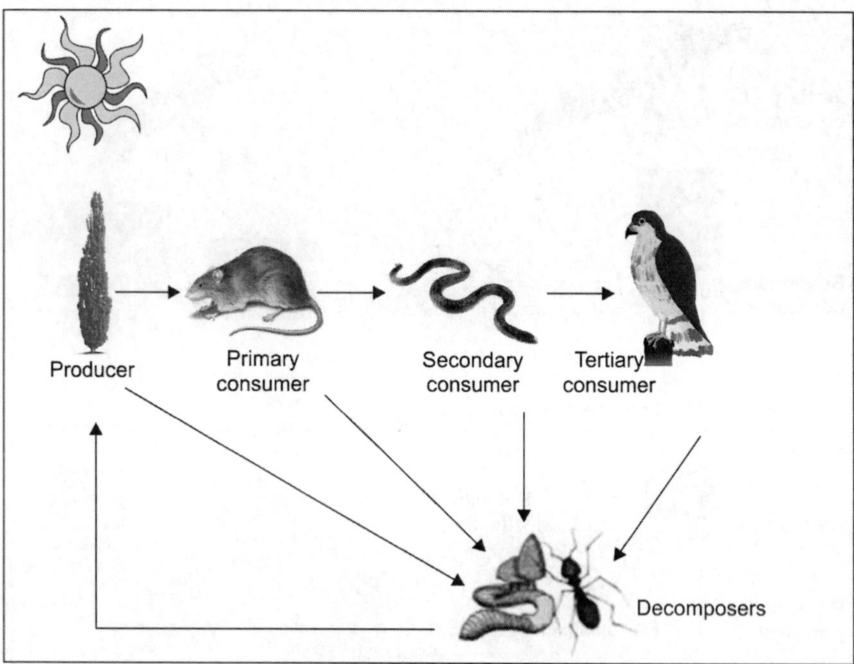

Fig. 5.7: Food chain

Water or Hydrological Cycle (Fig. 5.8)

The water cycle depicts the continuous flow of water on, above and below surface of earth. There is consistent water exchange occurs between air, land, sea and organisms. The mass of water remains same on earth over time but portioning of the water into major reservoirs of ice, fresh water, saline water and atmospheric water is variable depending on a wide range of climatic variables.

The hydrological cycle begins with evaporation of water from surface of ocean, ice and snow with solar energy and sublimate into water vapors.

- ***Evapotranspiration:*** This is the process under water vapors through plants and soil, and after reaching at upper layer of atmospheric air vapors condensed to form clouds. After rainfall again water reaches at surface of earth, then again two processes happen—one some of water evaporated back while rest of water seeped below soil and become groundwater.
- ***Groundwater:*** Groundwater again carries two processes some parts seeps its way to oceans, rivers and streams while rest of water evaporated back into atmosphere. Thus balance of water on the earth's surface flows to lakes, rivers and streams and all sources of waterflows towards oceans and again evaporation started.
- Hydrological cycle is the continuous and balanced process of evaporation, precipitation, transpiration, runoff water, condensation and infiltration.

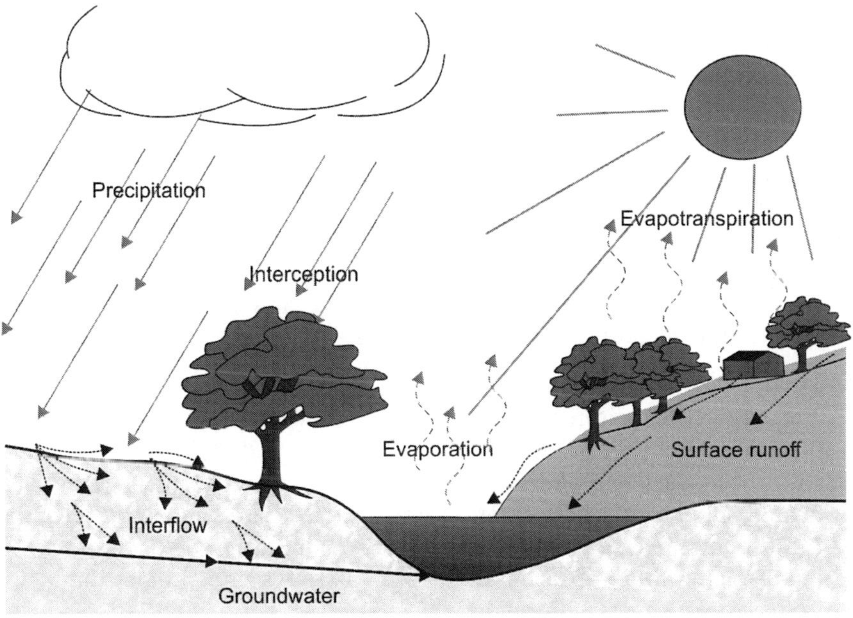

Fig. 5.8: Water or hydrologic cycle

Carbon Cycle (Fig. 5.9)

- Carbon is an organic compound and is a building block of both abiotic and biotic components.
- In an atmosphere carbon exists as CO_2 which is taken by producers (plants) through leaves for process of energy making, i.e. photosynthesis.

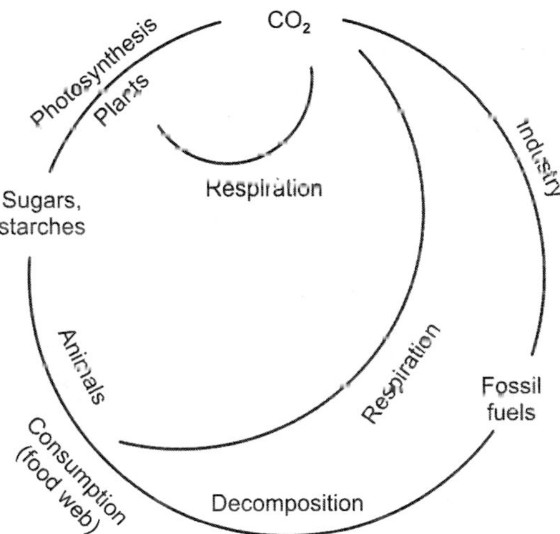

Fig. 5.9: Carbon cycle

- Photosynthesis is a process in which plants absorbed CO_2 and combine it with water absorbed from soil through roots in the presence of sunlight to form carbohydrates (energy).
- During photosynthesis plants produce energy for themselves for growth and development and during this process they release O_2 in atmosphere which is taken or absorbed by animals for respiration.
- Thus plants keep balance of atmospheric CO_2 and O_2.
- Herbivores animals feed on plants to produce energy for growth, CO_2 during respiration. Animals also return carbon to soil through excreta and when plant and animals died the carbon is released into soil through process and decomposition which completes environmental carbon cycle.

Oxygen Cycle (Fig. 5.10)

- The oxygen cycle is directly linked to carbon cycle through respiration and photosynthesis processes.
- Due to decreasing number of trees on earth's surface reducing oxygen level in atmosphere. Thus deforestation can result in serious consequences.
- Atmospheric oxygen also helps in maintaining ozone layer (O_3) of atmosphere which absorbs ultraviolet (UV) rays and protect mankind from adverse effects of these rays.

Nitrogen Cycle (Fig. 5.11)

- The defecated material of animals is broken down by worms and insects like ants and beetles.
- The insects and worms breakdown organic waste into smaller bits on which easily fungi and bacteria can survive.
- Thus these microscopic organisms decompose organic material and release nutrients in atmosphere and soil and these are back to plants through soil.
- Apparently, the dead bodies of animals also decomposed by micro-organisms and release nitrates into soil which fertilizes to plants and completed nitrogen cycle.

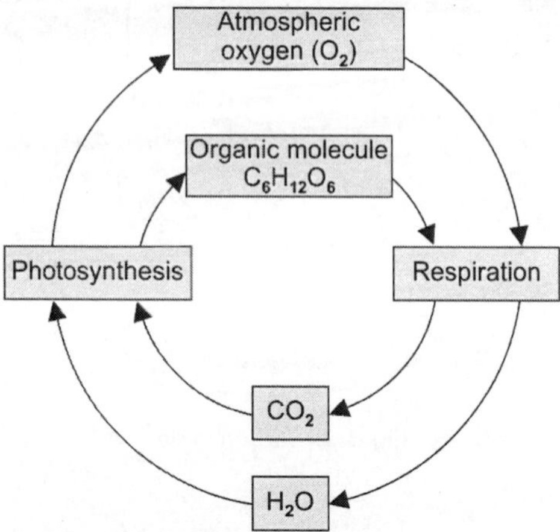

Fig. 5.10: Oxygen cycle

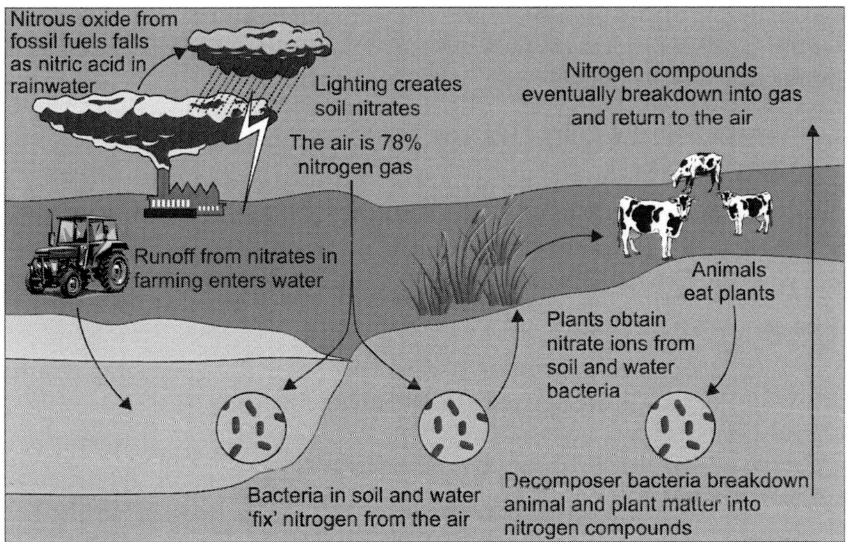

Fig. 5.11: Nitrogen cycle

- The nitrates are important nutrients for plants those help to plants in making new proteins which are transferred to carnivores' animals.

Phosphorus Cycle (Fig. 5.12)

- Phosphorus cycle describes the movement of phosphorus through the lithosphere, hydrosphere and biosphere.
- Soil microorganisms act as sinks and sources of available phosphorus in the biogeochemical cycle. However, the major transfers in the global cycle are driven by tectonic movements in geological time.
- On land, phosphorus is usually found in the water, soils and sediments.

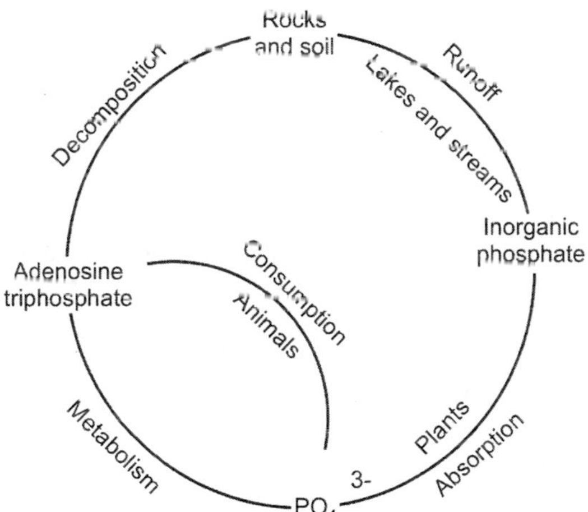

Fig. 5.12: Phosphorus cycle

- Weathering of rock phosphate gives out soil containing primary consumers from producers and runs to secondary consumers which they give out in the form of facial matter.

INTRODUCTION AND CHARACTERISTICS OF ALL TYPES OF ECOSYSTEMS

An ecosystem consists of both biotic and abiotic components living in specific type of ecosystem. However, all types of ecosystems can be categorized into two types: Terrestrial ecosystem and aquatic ecosystem.

Terrestrial Ecosystem

It refers to 'biome', i.e. the ecosystem which extends to a large geographic area and is land-based. The terrestrial ecosystem has following parts:

- Forest ecosystem
- Grassland ecosystem
- Desert ecosystem

Forest Ecosystem

Forests represent largest and ecologically complex systems which comprises of community of plants.

Definition: A forest ecosystem refers to an area dominated by trees and other woody plants, the richest source of biodiversity with both abiotic and biotic components.

Types of Forests

There are different types of forests exist in the world, ranging from tropical rain forests to the dense subpolar triage.

Tropical rainforests

- Hot and humid region of forest with annual rainfall approximately 2000–4500 mm
- Important in recycling of water
- Located at south and central America, western and central Africa, south east Asia, pacific ocean and certain islands of India.

Temperate forests:

- Cold in winter, warm and humid in summer with annual rainfall approximately 750–2000 mm
- Characterized by very fertile soil
- Found in western and central Europe, eastern Asia and eastern North America.

Coniferous forests

- Rich in coniferous trees, e.g. spruce, fir, pine, etc.
- Soil is acidic and humus rich
- Found in northern America, Europe and Asia.

The India has major four types of forests as follows:

1. ***Tropical rain forests***
   - Known as evergreen forests
   - Characterized by high rainfall approximately 1750–2000 mm

- Rich in plant diversity
- Have various medicinal plants
- Located in Kerala and Ladakh.

2. ***Temperate deciduous forests***
   - Consists of predominately broad leaf trees
   - Can be classified into two parts:
     i. ***Temperate forests:*** These forests can be categorized with moderate temperature and rainfall with chilly winters. The trees of forests drop leaves in autumn season.
     ii. ***Tropical forests:*** Forests with minimum temperature, moist and dry environment. The trees drop leaves in winter (December) season.
3. ***Moist deciduous forests***
   - Trees are tall with broad trunks
   - Dominated by sal and teak
   - Located in Himalayas, West Bengal, Sivalik Hills and Jammu.
4. ***Dry deciduous forests***
   - Rich in canopy trees
   - Located in Madhya Pradesh, Gujarat, Andhra Pradesh, Karnataka and Tamil Nadu, Andaman and Nikobar Islands.

Structure of Forests

The forest can be dividing into five layers as follows:

1. ***The canopy***
   - The very top layer of forest and comprised of tallest and oldest trees (150–200 feet)
   - Harshest layer directly exposed to sun, rainfall and atmospheric conditions
   - Animals live in this part of forest are mostly birds, tree frogs, snakes, lizards and hard bodied insects.
2. ***The understory***
   - Layer of forest just below the canopy
   - Comprised of growing trees
   - Have less exposure to sunlight thus trees grow at slow rate
   - Animals live in this part of forest are monkeys, raccoons, squirrels, tree mammals, frogs, caterpillars, butterflies and birds.
3. ***The shrub layer***
   - Next level down to understory
   - Dominated by less tall, woody plants. Most are shrubs
   - Animals live in this part are lichens, different kinds of insects, spiders, birds, snakes and lizards.
4. ***The herbaceous layer***
   - The herbaceous layer is 2nd last layer of forest
   - Comprised of seedlings and nonwoody plants
   - Contain mosses and flowering plants.
5. ***The forest floor***
   - The bottom and backbone layer of forest
   - Soil surface makeup of thick bed of dropped leaves.

Functions of Forest Ecosystem

- Acts as habitat for major flora and fauna
- Helps in conservation of biodiversity
- Reduce effects of global warming
- Protect water resources through less dispersion of water
- The high density of trees reduces soil erosion level
- Protect cultural dimensions of country.

Grassland Ecosystem

Grassland ecosystem occupied around 19% of earth's surface. The producers are mainly grasses, small trees and shrubs and soil is rich in nutrients.

Definition: Grasslands are the type of ecosystem where the dominant vegetation is grasses and shrubs. The important grassland is savanna in Africa.

Structure of Grassland

- Dominating vegetation is grass like structures.
- Covered up to 19 to 40% of earth's area
- Have nutrient rich fertile soil
- The important vegetation is termed as savanna.

Types of Grassland

Grassland is of two types:

1. ***Tropical grasslands:***
   - The important tropical grassland is savanna in Africa
   - Located in Africa, North America, Europe, Asia and Australia
   - Comprises of grasses and shrubs
   - Drought resistant and fire resistant
   - Habitat for giraffes, zebras, kangaroos, ground squirrels, snakes, lions, leopards and elephants
   - Climate is tropical wet and dry remains constant (hot) throughout the year
   - Soil is porous and rich with nutrients because of presence of decomposers.
2. ***Temperate grasslands***
   - Located on valdts of Africa, South America, Eurasia and North America
   - Grasses and flowering plants are dominant vegetations
   - A few trees like cottonwoods, oaks, and willows grow in temperate grassland
   - Have a low diversity in wild life. Provide habitat for animals like wolves, swift foxes as well as for birds like grouses, sparrows, hawks and owls
   - Climate is hot in summer and cold in winters
   - Soil is nutrient rich and fertile.

Functions of Grassland

- Habitat for producers, consumers and decomposers
- Composed of grasses such as wheat, provide grazing for livestock
- Consider as seedbed for ancestors of major cereal crops like wheat, rice, etc.
- Serve as breeding ground for thousands of bird species.

Desert Ecosystem

Desert ecology is the sum of the interactions between both biotic and abiotic processes in arid regions. It includes the interactions of plant, animal and bacterial populations in a desert habitat, ecosystem and community. The desert can be hot or cold and difficult for habitat.

Definition

A desert ecosystem is a community of organisms that live together in an environment that seems to be deserted wasteland or area with scanty rainfall.

Or

Deserts typically have harsh conditions due to unfavorable conditions like water scarcity, permanent frost and absence of soil thus harbors adverse living conditions.

Types of Desert Ecosystem

Hot desert

- Sahara is good example of hot desert.
- Scorching hot ground with little shades of plants.
- Shortage of water
- Scanty rainfall
- Plant grow those have tough skin, e.g. cactus
- Habitat is for reptiles, donkeys, camels, sheep and horses.

Cold desert

- Occur in temperature regions at higher latitudes
- Deserted rocky peaks of mountains
- Harsh environment
- Located in Ladakh
- Soil is mainly immature and alkaline
- Provide habitat to microbial communities.

Ice desert

- Another type of cold desert
- Uninhabited region composed of ice
- Located near north and south poles of the planet.

Aquatic Ecosystem

An aquatic ecosystem is group of interacting organisms with each other and water as an environment. Examples are ponds, lakes and rivers, etc.

Types of Aquatic Ecosystem

Pond ecosystem

- Most simple form of ecosystem
- Two phases:
  i. ***Wet phase***
     - The phytoplankton grow very rapidly
     - Zoo planktons thrive on it.

  ii. ***Dry phase***
     - The population of phytoplankton get reduced
     - Thus affects the population of zoo planktons.

Lake ecosystem

- Permanent form of pond ecosystem
- *Algae* species dominate in this ecosystem and zoo planktons feed on *Algae* species to get energy.
- The phytoplankton and the zoo plankton utilize dissolved oxygen and sunlight which penetrates in water.

River ecosystem

- Most dynamic ecosystem
- Flowing water ecosystems or fresh water ecosystem
- Fresh water is utilized by humans
- In this ecosystem fish species are abundant.

Marine ecosystem

- Widest and maximum extended ecosystem
- In this organisms receive sunlight which penetrates in water
- Below surface in deep layers plankton do not receive sunlight.

ASSESSMENT

Essay Type Questions

1. Define ecosystem. Discuss in detail about components of ecosystem.
2. Describe in detail about food chain and food web.
3. Discuss with suitable examples about energy flow and material cycling in ecosystem.
4. Describe various types of ecosystem.

Multiple Choice Questions

1. The term 'ecology' was coined by:
   (a) Earnst Hackel (b) Einstein
   (c) AG Tansley (d) None of the above
2. Transfer of energy from one organism to another in an ecosystem takes place in a:
   (a) Linear manner (b) Hierarchical manner
   (c) Discrete manner (d) Cyclic manner
3. Which one of the following describe best to term 'ecosystem'?
   (a) A community of organisms interacting with one another
   (b) The part of earth inhabited by living organisms
   (c) A community of organisms together with the environment in which they live
   (d) The flora and fauna of geographical area
4. Biotic component of ecosystem involves:
   (a) Living organisms (b) Nonliving organisms
   (c) Both (a) and (b) (d) None of the above
5. 'Omnivorous' is the term used for organisms who consume:
   (a) Only plants (b) Only other animals
   (c) Both plants and animals (d) None of the above

Fill in the Blanks

6. The energy flow in ecosystem occurs through ___________ and ___________.
7. The building block of abiotic and biotic components of ecosystem is ___________.
8. The photosynthesis process needs chlorophyll, CO_2 and _________ for completion.
9. The oxygen cycle is directly linked to carbon cycle through two processes known as ___________ and ___________.
10. The canopy is the ___________ layer of forest.

ANSWERS

1. a	2. d	3. c	4. a
5. c	6. Food web, Food chain		7. Carbon
8. H_2O	9. Respiration, Photosynthesis		10. First

Current Environmental Issues

CHAPTER

6

Learning Objectives

After the end, the students will be able to:

- Define population explosion and effects of population explosion.
- Describe effects of population explosion on environment and human health.
- Define urbanization and effects of urbanization on environment and human health.
- Define acid rain and its ill effects.
- Define global warming and effects on environment.
- Define climate and its effect on environment.

HUMAN POPULATION AND ENVIRONMENT

Population includes total number of persons inhabiting an area, country or city. Population includes study of population statistics and trends. The demographic process context put huge impact on environmental context.

Distribution of Population

It indicates the pattern where people live and can be categorized into sparsely populated areas and densely populated areas.

Factors Affecting Distribution of Population

- ***Physical factors:*** Landforms, agriculture, vegetation soils and water supplies.
- ***Climatic conditions:*** The moderate climate includes refreshing and pleasant environment contributes in inclined and dense population. The areas with too hot and too cold environments are sparsely populated areas.
- ***Natural resources:*** The lands wealthy in natural resources like coal, forest, minerals, water etc. favors population density. For instance Europe, Bihar and West Bengal are highly populated areas.
- ***Soils:*** The soil rich in fertility is backbone of substantially high yield per hector in agriculture thus these type of soils supports population density. For example East and South Asian Regions and Northern Plains of India are densely populated areas.
- ***Means of transportation and communication***
  - Highly developed means of air, surface and water add to density of population in particular region because there the people can manage and carry on agricultural, commercial as well as industrial activities.
  - Economic factors resources, accessibility, diseases and pests, stages of economical development etc.

- ***Politicalfactors:*** Stability of government, political scope for development, efficient bureaucracy, restrictions of international boundaries etc.

Types of Population on the Basis of Growth

There are three types of population:

1. ***Rapidly growing population:*** It is a population which has high birth rate and low death rate, so there are more numbers of young individuals in the population.
2. ***Stationary population:*** It is a population which has equal birth rate and death rates, so population shows zero population growth.
3. ***Declining population:*** It is a population which has higher death rate than birth rate, so the population has more numbers of older individuals.

Population Growth

Population in the world is currently (2017) growing at a rate of around 1.11% per year (down from 1.13% in 2016). The current average population change is estimated at around 80 million per year. This means that world population will continue to grow in the 21st century, but at a slower rate compared to the recent past. World population has doubled (100% increase) in 40 years from 1959 (3 billion) to 1999 (6 billion). It is now estimated that it will take a further 39 years to increase by another 50%, to become 9 billion by 2038. (Statistics taken from world meter).

The factors considered in population growth are:

- Change in population can be measured both in terms of absolute numbers and in percentage.
- Natural growth rate of population can be measured as the ratio of the difference between births and deaths by population to the total population at the beginning of the period and multiplying it with hundred.

$$\frac{\text{Births - Deaths}}{\text{Total population at the beginning}} \times 100$$

- The negative rates of natural increase results from an excess of deaths over births. Positive rates of natural increase results from an excess of births over deaths.
- Basic component of population growth are fertility, mortality and migration. These three components are measured to calculate change in magnitude of population.

Rates to Measure Population Growth

The change in population of any area can be measured through two components, i.e. fertility and mortality.

Fertility

Fertility refers to the occurrence of births in required area. This can be measured through following rates:

- ***Crude birth rate:*** It is the number of live births on per thousand births in a year and brings out exact rate at which the population increases through birth.

$$\text{Crude birth rate} = \frac{\text{Number of live births in a year}}{\text{Population (mid-year)}}$$

- ***Fertility ratio:*** It is expressed in terms of children below 5 years of age per 1000 females of reproductive age group.

$$\text{Fertility ratio} = \frac{\text{Population of children below 5 years}}{\text{Female population between 15 to 49 years}} \times 1000$$

Mortality

Mortality includes the number of deaths occurred in particular country in single year. This can be measured as following:

- ***Crude death rate (CDR):*** It is measured as the number of deaths per 1000 estimated mid-year population in one year in a given place.

$$\text{Crude death rate} = \frac{\text{Number of death during the year}}{\text{Mid-year population}} \times 1000$$

- ***Infant mortality rate (IMR):*** It measures the probability of death in the first year of life are the sum of neonatal mortality rate (from birth to age 28 days) and postneonatal mortality rate (from 1 to 11 months of age).
- ***Child mortality rate (CMR) or under 5 mortality rate (U5MR):*** It refers to deaths from birth up to a child's 5th birthday. Each rate is calculated as number of deaths in the specific age group per 1000 live births.

Population Explosion

Population explosion can be defined as the electrifying and accelerated growth in population over past 100 years in world history. It is associated with high birth rate and low death rate which also can be considered as major causes for population explosion. But in present the rate of growth has been declined a little bit over the recent past few years.

According to United Nations projections, the world population will be between 7.9 billion and 10.9 billion by 2050. Much of increase is taking place in developing countries as compared to industrialized nations.

In India population explosion can be considered as curse because it is continuously damaging to development of country.

Population change = (births + immigrations) (deaths + emigrations)

Causes of Population Explosion Globally

The causes of population can be:

- Increase in birth rate due to appropriate medical provisions.
- Decrease in death rate due to better medical facilities and advancement in medical techniques.
- Immigration to developed countries for better opportunities like job, life quality, natural disasters etc.

As a developing country India may be having following reasons for population explosion:

Increase in Birth Rate

In terms of population India is at second to China as well as globally. As per 2017 statistics Indian population is equal to 17.86% of total world population and density is 452 per km^2. The median age in India is 26.9 years. In 2017 the yearly population change in India is 1.18% and fertility rate is 2.45.

Reasons of increase in birth rate

- ***Poverty:*** More than 300 million Indians are below poverty line thus this is thinking that more children more hand to earn. Apparently, because of lack of food and medical facilities the number of children produce may not survive all.
- ***Religious belief, traditions and cultural norms:*** Because of high illiteracy rate most of people still stick to historical belief that God said, 'go and produce, so we are doing same.' In addition the preference of son edged over daughters results in giving births to more children. In rural areas still child marriage is a norm contributed in increased population.

Decrease in Death Rate

Various factors contribute in decrease in death rate as follows:

- ***Control of diseases:*** The advances made in medical sciences have reduced incidence rate of diseases and formulation and implementation of preventive vaccines resulted in decreased death rate.
- ***Decrease in infant mortality rate:*** The advancements in public health sector and maternal and child health sector have declined infant mortality rate.
- ***Increase in life expectancy:*** Due to big improvement in living conditions, hygiene and sanitation habits and health education has significantly increased life expectancy globally.
- ***Improvement in agriculture:*** Due to inclining in technological measures the agricultural production hiked to fulfill need of food for all and thus results in better nutrition conditions which declined malnutrition diseases and deaths due to starvation.

Effects of Population Explosion

- ***Over population:*** The increase in numbers of live births will increase crowd result in over population or congestion on land
- ***Unemployment:*** In developing countries due to overpopulation the opportunities for daily living earnings are reducing day-by-day and creating an army of unemployed people.
- ***Poverty:*** The giant problem of high birth rate is associated with poverty. The low income is both reason and effect of population explosion as well as vice-versa.
- ***Illiteracy:*** Low education rate cause lack of awareness regarding birth control measures resulting in inclined population. On the other side, in poor families couples produce more children to increase hands for earning.
- ***Poor health status:*** Due to inadequate availability of food and shelter causes malnutrition and associated diseases reduces health status of country population.
- ***Economy:*** The demand for consumption should never exceed production or resource limit otherwise causes a big stumbling block in economical development of country.

- ***Environment hazard:*** The crowding of people create hazardous consequences for environment by various means like increase in waste, deforestation, industrialization and inclined pollution, etc.

Effects of Population Explosion of Environment

The rapid growth of birth rate is putting negative strain on our natural environment. For instance developed countries are damaging to environment because of mass industrialization and developing countries are under pressure to meet with demands of economy are damaging environment as well.

The major consequences are:

- ***Pollution:*** Due to increase in number of people will incline the amount of refusal and garbage causes degradation of environment. Along with this increase in number of use of automobiles causes smoke and gas pollution damaging natural habitat.
- ***Deforestation:*** The overpopulation has created scarcity of residential land thus people are converting forests and agricultural land into residential areas increasing number of deforestation and reducing number of trees and plants. Thus, it has increased soil erosion, floods and extinction of various animal species due to lack of habitat which is harming to natural food chain.
- ***Fresh water availability:*** The increased demand of freshwater created lack of resources of water. As well as deforestation has reduced rainfall and excessive use of ground reduced table of water below soil which will be a huge challenge in front of human species in near future.
- ***Natural resources:*** Over consumption of non-renewable resources like coal, petroleum, fossil fuels is leading towards early deduction of boom of natural resources which can create major consequences for our next generations.
- ***Global warming:*** The increase in number of persons has also increased use of vehicles which emits harmful gases in environment. The rising number of industries, cutting of trees, use of other technical equipments is continuously contributing in increase of environmental temperature due to harm to ozone layer called global warming.

Control Measures

Population explosion is a huge stumbling block in development of any country like in India. Since this problem is getting intense day-by-day, the following measures can be use to keep check on increase in population:

- ***Rise in per capita income:*** Government should take measures to increase per capita income and employment opportunities to make earning easy for daily needs then couples will not desire more children to increase earning hands for fulfillment of family needs.
- ***Urbanization and industrialization:*** Urbanization should be encouraged which will rise level of life of people and create awareness among people regarding short family norms. Whereas increased number of industries will blossom with employment opportunities for youth.
- ***Late marriage:*** The making strict ethics and laws against child marriage and increase in minimum marriage age will reduce birth rate of country.

- ***Lowering infant mortality rate:*** The widespread vaccination and accurate provision of maternal and child health services will reduce infant mortality rate and help in increase of sense of security regarding children's loss among parents.
- ***Literacy level:*** The increase in literacy level will help in moving belief of having children as God's wish and poverty which will decrease birth rate in country.
- ***Women education and employment:*** In India, still there are few families and communities who do not believe in female education and employment. The awareness regarding this will create acceptance of short family norm.
- ***Family planning facilities:*** The family planning centers for awareness and provision of facilities should be placed at rural as well as urban areas to control birth rate.
- The government should raise incentives both monetary and real to encourage family planning.
- ***Legislation:*** The government should enact laws for lowering the birth rate. For example, China adopted a policy of 'we are two and we have one' to reduce policy.

■ HUMAN HEALTH AND URBANIZATION

In the ancient time, the major environmental issues were related to wild-life, endangered species, pollution and human health hazards due to agricultural impacts. But in present the major issue is urbanization as threat to environment.

Urbanization is the evolution of cities, industrialization and commercialization in developed parts of country.

Urbanization is an inevitable phenomenon that accompanies the development of a country.

Definition of Urbanization

Urbanization can be defined as the inclining population in cities and towns in comparison to villages and remote areas. Urbanization occur because of immigration of workers to cities from villages with evolution of industries and manufacturing hubs as well as more opportunities of jobs. The high and facilitated living standard also attracts to people from rural to urban area.

Or

Urbanization is the growing number of people in a society living in urban areas, or cities. Urbanization means increased spatial scale and density of settlement as well as business and other activities in the area. Urban areas tend to attract businesses because of their large and dense population. This in turn draws more people to the area, working in a kind of circular process.

Or

Urbanization is defined as the process of human movement and centralization towards and into cities and urban areas with the associated industrialization, urban sprawl and lifestyle that brings.

The Census of Urbanization in India

- As per 2001 census in India urbanization was identified by two ways:
  1. ***Statutory towns:*** These are the places with a municipality, corporation, cantonment board or notified town area committee etc., e.g. Shimla (Municipal Corporation).
  2. ***Census towns:*** These are the places which satisfied following three criteria:
     a. A minimum population of 5000
     b. At least, 75% of the male main working population engaged in non-agricultural pursuits
     c. A density of population is at least 400 per sq. km.
- The total urban population in the country as per census 2011 is more than 377 million constituting 31.16% of the total population. This may happen because of rapid migration of population
- Growth of cities depends upon two factors:
  1. Enlargement of urban centers
  2. Emergence of new towns.

Urban Settlement According to Census of India

The urban settlement can be classified into six categories on the basis of characteristics of population size as per census.

- ***City:*** Urban population with more than one lakh is considered as city.
- ***Town:*** The area with population of less than 1 lakh is termed as town.
- Urban Agglomeration (UA)
  - The population should be more than 20000
  - Must consist of at least one statutory town
  - A town adjoining urban outgrowths
  - Two or more contiguous towns
  - A city and one or more adjoining towns with their outgrowths together forming a contiguous spread.
- ***Out growth (OGs):*** An out growth is a viable unit such as a village that is clearly identifiable in terms of its boundaries and location. For example, university campus, railway colony etc.
- As per census in 2011, in India the number was of:
  - Towns: 2774
  - Statutory towns: 4041
  - Census towns: 3894
  - Urban agglomerations: 475
  - Out growths: 981

Impacts of Urbanization on Environment

- Slums and its consequences of overcrowding
- Lack of sanitation
- Poverty, illiteracy and unemployment
- Increased crime
- Deforestation

- Pollution and global warming
- Increase in slums
- Increase in diseases like infection salmonella typhus, hepatitis, HIV, AIDS, etc.
- Evolution of slums due to overcrowding.

ACID RAIN

Acid rain is a type of rain with more acidic water than normal range because of more atmospheric pollution. Acid rain alters the climate, soil, water resources concentration and life cycles of plants and animals. The major contents of acid rain are sulfur dioxide and nitrogen dioxide. pH is the scale measuring the amount of acid in the water and liquid. The pH scale ranges from 0 to 14 with a lower pH being more acidic while a high pH is alkaline; seven is neutral. Normal rain water is slightly acidic and has a pH range of 5.3–6.0. Acid deposition is anything below that range. It is also important to note that the pH scale is logarithmic and each whole number on the scale represents a 10-fold change.

Definition

Acid rain can be defined as precipitation of relatively high concentrations of acid-forming chemicals mixes with rain water, as the pollutants from coal smoke, chemical manufacturing, and smelting, that have been released into the atmosphere and combined with water vapor: harmful to the environment.

Causes of Acid Rain

Natural Sources

- Volcanoes
- Fossil fuel combustion
- Dispersion of chemicals in environment through wind
- Natural disaster disruption.

Man-made Sources

- Industrialization and industrial revolution
- Automobiles
- Burning of coal
- Deforestation.

Types of Acid Rain

Acid rain has two types:

1. ***Wet deposition:*** Wet deposition refers to acidic rain, fog, and snow. As this acidic water flows over and through the ground, it affects a variety of plants and animals.
2. ***Dry deposition:*** Dry deposition refers to acidic gases and particles. About half of the acidity in the atmosphere falls back to earth through dry deposition.

Formation of Acid Rain

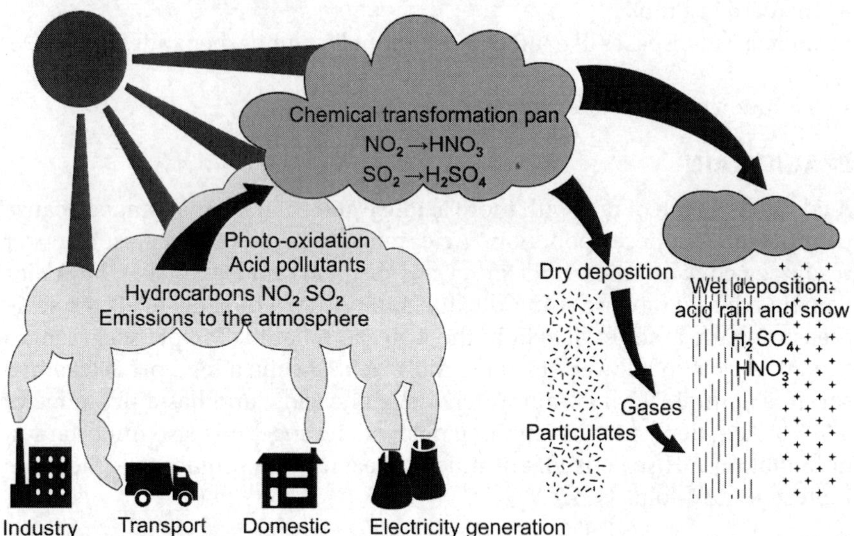

Effects of Acid Rain

The effects of acid rain can be divided into three categories:
1. On non-living things
2. On living things
3. On soil

On Non-living Things

- The Taj Mahal in Agra, suffering from sulfur dioxide, sulfuric acid and other fumes pollutants released from Mathura refinery.
- Acid rain causes extensive damage to building, statues, bridges and structural materials of marble, limestone, etc.

On Living Things

- ***Human health:*** The sulfur dioxide and nitrogen oxide gases causes respiratory diseases like asthma, chronic bronchitis, etc.
- Tiny particles cause difficulty in breathing for humans and animals and also lead to permanent lung damage.

On Water Animals

Acid rain increases the acidity of lakes and rivers which is directly affect the aquatic ecosystem.

On Trees and Soil

- Acid rain dissolves all the nutrients and the useful minerals for the tree to grow.
- Weakens the process of photosynthesis.
- According to modern researchers, acid rain leaches potassium, calcium, magnesium, etc. essential elements from the top of soil and when soil is contaminated, cereal (arable) production crops.

- Acids activate aluminium from the soil which leaches into water and fish die. Drinking water is contaminated.

Solution of Acid Rain

- Fit scrubbers into factory's chimneys which are chemical filters that remove impurities such as sulfur from smoke.
- Cars can be fitted with special converters which remove dangerous chemicals.
- Governments need to spend more money on pollution control.
- Governments need to invest in researching different ways to produce energy.

■ CLIMATE CHANGES

The changes in average weather for a particular location are termed as climate changes.

The changes may be due to natural processes and human activities which causes alternation regular and normal climate of place.

Definition

A change in global or regional climate patterns, in particular a change apparent from the mid to late 20th century onwards and attributed largely to the increased levels of atmospheric carbon dioxide produced by the use of fossil fuels.

Causes of Climate Change

The causes behind the changes in climate can be categorized in two parts:

1. Natural causes
2. Man-made causes

Natural Causes

The climate of earth influenced through natural changes and disasters like volcanic eruption, ocean currents etc.

Man-made Causes (Anthropogenic Causes)

- ***Greenhouse gases:*** The activities of human are increasing emission of gases those are causing ozone depleting gases in environment and increasing temperature on planet.
- ***Cryogenic processes:*** The processes of permafrost, glaciations, defrosting and deglaciations are known as cryogenic processes. The recent evidences have shown that the ice sheets of Antarctica, Greenland, and Baffin Island etc. are beating, thinning and melting.
- ***Black carbon:*** It is solid produced from incomplete combustion of carbon containing materials and responsible for more than 30% of recent warming in Arctic region.
- ***Greenhouse effects:***
  - The solar energy maintains earth's climate and weather and heat's the earth's surface. When the surface of earth heats it emits certain gases like CO_2, water, vapors back in the environment and these gases are known

as greenhouse gases and greenhouse gases effect results in increase of temperature of earth's surface due to atmospheric trap energy of gases.

- The major six greenhouse gases are CO_2, CH_4, N_2O, hydrofluorocarbon, Perfluorocarbon and sulfur hexafluoride, water vapors.
- The increase in concentration of greenhouse gases may increase absorption of radiations at surface of earth.

Effects of Climate Change

- The climate change can severely affect human societies, agriculture and the natural ecosystem, terrestrial and aquatic ecosystem those are hub of natural sources.
- The high temperatures of earth will cause melting of glaciers results in concentration of environmental methane hydrate and CO_2 that will increase temperature of earth.
- The climate warm forced out to various species of plants and animals from their natural habitat places.
- The increased climate temperature causes wild fire disasters.
- The climate change will alter the cycle of agricultural and forestry crops and plantation.
- The rising sea level due to glaciers melting severely affect coastline resulting in floods.
- The increase in global temperature will aid in outbreak of diseases.

Effects of Climate Change in India

- Coastal inundation and therefore, resulting population displacement.
- Fall in crop fields resulting in food insecurity. It is estimated that every 1°C increase in temperature is likely to lead to 5–10% reduction in yields of some crops.
- Increase in bacterial infection, e.g. vector born diseases and respiratory diseases.

Indian Government's Efforts to Manage Climate Changes

Prime Minister's National Action Plan for Climate Changes (NAPCC).

Name of Mission Nodal agencies initiated by Government of India and Nodal are as follows:

- National Solar Mission
- National Mission on Sustainable Habitat
- National Water Mission
- National Mission for Sustaining the Himalayan Ecosystem
- National Mission for Green India
- National Mission for Sustainable Agriculture
- National Mission for Strategic Knowledge for Climate Change
- National Green Tribunal (NGT) Act.

OZONE DEPLETION

- Ozone is a gas that is naturally present in atmosphere.
- The 90% of ozone present in stratosphere, a region begins about 9 miles above earth's surface and is known as ozone layer.

- The rest 10% is found in troposphere.
- The ozone layer acts as protective covering of earth from sun's harmful ultraviolet rays and ozone depletion will cause increased introduction of UV rays on earth surface causing increase in temperature.
- The ozone depletion is caused by greenhouse gases present in atmosphere emitted by earth's surface with heating.
- Chlorofluorocarbons (CFCs) and other halogenated ozone depleting substances (ODS) are mainly responsible for man-made chemical ozone depletion.

Effects of Ozone Depletion

- The depletion of ozone layer will cause excessive exposure of humans to ultraviolet radiations will cause skin cancer, sun burns, weakening of immune system etc.
- The overexposure of ultraviolet rays to plants will harm photosynthesis procedure resulting in poor growth of plants and poor agricultural crops.
- The high temperature will alter the marine life. The exposure of harmful rays will also photosynthesis process of planktons that will alter the marine food chain.

Solutions to Ozone Depletion

- ***Desist from using pesticides:*** The reduction in use of pesticides will help in get rid of problem of ozone depletion and encourage using ecofriendly methods to treat weed and pests in agricultural fields.
- ***Discourage driving of private vehicles:*** The easiest technique to minimize ozone depletion is to limit the number of vehicles on the road. These vehicles emit a lot of greenhouse gases that eventually form smog, a catalyst in the depletion of ozone layer.
- ***Utilize environmentally friendly cleaning products:*** Most household cleaning products are loaded with harsh chemicals that find way to the atmosphere, eventually contributing to degradation of the ozone layer. Use natural and environmentally friendly cleaning products to arrest this situation.
- Prohibit the use of harmful nitrous oxide.

■ GLOBAL WARMING

The temperature of earth is increasing day-by-day refers as global warming. The changes in natural climate and certain man-made activities are contributing in temperature around the globe.

Definition

An increase in the average temperature of the earth's atmosphere and ocean, especially a sustained increase sufficient to cause climatic change is known as global warming.

Impacts of Global Warming

- ***Extreme weather patterns:*** The scientists believe that global warming will cause climate change resulting in extreme changes in weather:
  - More hurricanes and drought
  - Longer spells of dry heat and intense rain.
- ***Rising sea levels and super storms:*** The increase in temperature on earth's surface causes melting of glaciers and increased sea level resulting in floods and will cause death of various land and marine species. Global warming may spawn more super storms resulting in destruction in life and materials.
- ***Ocean acidification***
  - More CO_2 in the atmosphere means more CO_2 in the water of ocean.
  - Atmospheric CO_2 is dissolved in the ocean which becomes more acidic.
  - The resulting changes in the chemistry of the oceans disrupts the ability of plants and animals in the sea to make shells and skeleton of calcium carbonate, while dissolving shells already formed.
- ***Global dimming:*** Clouds are formed when water droplets are seeded by airborne particles such as pollen. Polluted air results in clouds with larger number of droplets than unpolluted clouds. This makes clouds more effective. More of the sun's heat and energy is therefore reflected back into space. This reduction of heat reaching the earth is known as global warming.

ASSESSMENT

Essay Type Questions

1. Define population explosion. Describe in detail about causes and effects of population explosion.
2. Define acid rain and its effects on human health.
3. Discuss in detail about ozone depletion.
4. Define climate change on earth. Explain in detail about its effects on life on earth.
5. Discuss about reasons of climate changes globally and at national level.
6. Define urbanization and its effect on natural environment.

Biodiversity: Conservation and Importance

CHAPTER 7

Learning Objectives

At the end of study of this unit students will be able to:
- Define biodiversity.
- Classified levels and divisions of biodiversity.
- Describe facts, importance and threats to biodiversity.
- Explain about conservation methods of biodiversity.

BIODIVERSITY

Variety of Life on Earth

Biodiversity is variations in species or ecosystem variation within an area, biome or planet. Biodiversity is more than just species. It includes genetic variations.

Definition

The term refers to describe the number, variation or diversity of living organisms on earth.

Or

Biological diversity in an environment is indicated by number of different species of plants and animals.

Levels of Biodiversity

Biodiversity has mainly three levels:
1. ***Genetic diversity:*** It refers to variation of genes exists within a species. It represents the inherited variation within population for instance different breeds of dogs within same species.
2. ***Ecological diversity:*** It points towards variations of ecosystem natural communities and habitats. In nature the variety of methods of interaction within species and environment.
3. ***Species diversity:*** It refers to number of species in a site or habitat.

Division of Biodiversity as per Location

- ***Terrestrial biodiversity:*** The variation of species is highest near the equator due to warm climate and high primary productivity.
- ***Marine biodiversity:*** It refers to the highest species diversity along coasts in the western pacific where sea surface temperature is highest and mid latitudinal band in all oceans located.

Hotspots of Biodiversity in India

Biodiversity in India can be divided into two hotspots or zones:

1. ***Eastern Himalaya's biodiversity:*** The Himalayan region is richest center of diversity. It comprises of Nepal, Bhutan, states of east and north, east India and south-western China. It is formed of a distinct floral region contains, 5800 plant species roughly 2000 (36%) of which are endemic and also have 55 rare species of plants, e.g. pitcher plant.
2. ***Western Ghats's biodiversity:*** The western Ghats region also known as Monsoon Mountains covered area of 6 states of India like Maharashtra-Gujarat border, Goa, Kerala, Karnataka, Tamil Nadu and Kanayakumari. These rainy mountains have large forests which comprises of 5000 species of plants, 315 species of vertebrates, 140 species of mammals, 510 species of birds, 260 species of reptiles, 180 species of amphibians and 104 species of fish. This area of India is great source of water and oxygen with hot climate thus provide favorable conditions to flora and fauna.

Facts about Biodiversity

The Indian biodiversity encompasses large number of species approximately 1.7 million having following facts:

- The biodiversity is more abundant in tropical ecosystem as compared to temperate and boreal ecosystem. Thus tropical rain forests give birth to huge variety of species.
- The invertebrates group (animals without backbone, e.g. insects, scorpions, etc.) have variations of species as compared to others.
- There is also huge biodiversity among microscopic organisms like bacteria and protozoa.

Importance of Biodiversity

Biodiversity plays vital role in health of people and ecosystem. The important values are following:

- ***Economy:*** The various species aided in benefitting economy of country through their special character like silkworm produces specific fiber and certain species helps in making drugs, special food chains contributing in inclining country's economy.
- ***Variety of food:*** Due to abundance in variety of species it creates variety in food web in both vegetarian and nonvegetarian as well as help in maintaining natural food chain.
- ***Health sciences:*** Biodiversity has contributed as a stepping stone in pharmaceutical industry and health sciences in invention of various drugs for treatments and prevention of hazardous diseases.
- ***Ecological services:*** The variation on earth's natural geobiography has everything from cleaning of water to providing fresh oxygen for survival. It also absorbs harmful contents present in environment to prevent disasters.
- ***Adaptations:*** Biodiversity allows for ecosystem to adjust and adapt during natural disasters like flooding, forest fire and droughts, etc. as well as create environmental adaptations for changes occur in natural climate of species for balance in nature.

Threats to Biodiversity

Extinction and changes are natural part of life on earth. Over the history various species went extinct and came into origin due to consistent changes in ecosystem and habitat.

At present, the vital threat to biodiversity is accelerated rate of extinction of various unique species on earth because of unnatural human activities.

These activities of humans put direct ill effect on various species through following:

- ***Extinction:*** This is ending of species of plant or animal. The tragic environmental calamites are creating extinction of valuable species on earth. According a report issued by the International Union for Conservation of Nature (IUCN) Red List in 2014, 15 species of birds, 12 species of mammals, and 18 species of reptiles and amphibians have joined the critically endangered list. The most endangered species are red panda, tigers, crocodile, etc.
- ***Habitat degradation/loss:*** This is the reason of extinction of various species globally; deforestation due to population explosion is creating halt to natural habitat of distinct species. Due to fragmentation of land causes difficulty in carrying pollens through various animals decreasing plant species.
- ***Over exploitation:*** Because of industrial advancements in health sciences demands more animals for experimentation as well as over use of pesticides in agricultural fields causing extinction of species. For example production of monocrop has created feeding problems for various animals and birds leading towards their end of species because of scarcity of food.
- ***Climate change:*** The abrupt changes in climate increases migration of birds and animals, this creates problems in food web and food chain resulting in end of various species.
- ***Pollution:*** The introduction of various harmful and chemical contents in environment because of high degree of pollution created by humans is creating difficult time of survival for birds, animals and plants.
- ***Poaching of wild life:*** Hunting of wild as well as marine life endangered the existence of various species. The major factors behind poaching of animals is increase in food, pharmaceutical and fashion industries.
- ***Exotic species:*** The experimentation and hibernation of breed almost kill the native species and caused various gene mutations resulting in characteristic changes in animals. Sometimes, these experiments results in birth of daggered animals.

■ BIODIVERSITY CONSERVATION

Humans are dependent upon nature for everything like growth, development, food, shelter, health, cultural diversity, etc. and biodiversity plays vital role in existence of human species.

Thus the protection and preservation of natural diversity became essential as well as moral duty of humans.

Conservation efforts can be grouped into the following two categories:

1. ***In situ conservation:*** This is also called on-site conservation of biodiversity. This process includes protection of species in their natural habitat without any manipulation and migration, e.g. protected habitat of forests and sea.
2. ***Ex situ conservation:*** This is also called off-site conservation of biodiversity. This process includes protection of plants and animals outside of their natural habitat under artificial conditions thus include manipulation of natural environment.

In situ Conservation of Biodiversity (On-site Conservation)

Protection of habitat: The main objective of in situ conservation is the protection of habitats in representative ecosystem. The ministry of environment and forests, Government of India has proposed 15.67 (4.7%) million hectares of geographical area for conservation of biodiversity in their natural locations like forests. Apparently, 21 wetlands, 30 mangrove areas and 4 coral reef areas have been identified for intensive conservation by government of India.

This project includes following steps:

- ***National parks and sanctuaries:*** The government of India has delivered protection to natural habitat of species by grounding them national sanctuaries and national parks where natural habitat is maintained by various agencies without any manipulation. The major sanctuaries in India are:
  - The Jim Corbett Tiger Reserve - Uttaranchal
  - Kanha National Park - Madhya Pradesh
  - Bandhugarh National Park - Madhya Pradesh
  - Ranthambor National Park - Sawai Madhopur
  - Gir National Park - Sasangir, Gujarat
  - Kanjiranga National Park - Assam

  The India's richest and unique biodiversity is conserved at Ladakh in Himalayas, known as India National Park and Wild Life Sanctuaries. Presently, India has 96 national parks and 500 sanctuaries.
- ***Biosphere reserves:*** The UNESCO's Man and the Biosphere Programme (MAB) include 13 biodiversity conservation ecosystems. The main functions of biosphere reserves are following:
  - ***Conservation:*** The preservation of different types of ecosystems and landscapes along with their genetic species, flora and fauna.
  - ***Development:*** To encourage traditional resources use for promotion of sustainable cultural, social and ecological development.
  - ***Scientific research monitoring and education:*** The exchange of information regarding conservation of biodiversity at local, national and global level.
- ***Species oriented projects:*** Certain species have been declared in need of specific and direct protection efforts, e.g. tigers, elephants and crocodiles. Under this view following projects have been implemented:

- ***Project tiger:*** A success in species conservation. In Indian forests the population of tigers is drastically declining due to poaching. The project tiger was initiated in 1973 with objective of preservation and rescuing of this species from extinction. The land with area 37,671 km^2 has been projected for this project.
- ***Project elephant:*** To protect wild elephant's population in their natural habitat 12 states were aided under this project in February, 1992.
- ***Crocodile breeding and management project:*** The three endangered species the fresh water crocodile, the salt water crocodile and rare gharial, have been protected through sanctuaries and national parks. This project was started in 1970 with FAO-UNDP assistance. The government of India launched project for crocodile breeding in 1975 at Odisha extended to Rajasthan, Madhya Pradesh, Maharashtra, Bihar and Nagaland.
- ***Sacred forests and sacred lakes:*** The few forests and lakes have been declared as sacred to protect wild life and marine life from hunting. For example in India certain forest patches located in Karnataka, Maharashtra, Kerala, etc. are protected by tribal communities form hunting by people. Apparently, certain lakes in India and Asia have been declared as sacred to protect marine life, the best example of this is Khecheopalri Lake in Sikkim.

Ex Situ Conservation (Off-site Conservation)

The protection of biodiversity by providing artificial habitat by following means:

- ***Botanical Garden, Zoos:*** The various agencies have implanted botanical gardens, zoos, medicinal plant parks to preserve species by artificial habitat. The best example for this is the 200 years old 'The Indian Botanical Garden' in Howrah (West Bengal). Recently, The Botanical Garden of Indian Republic has been established at Noida in 2002. The main objectives of these gardens are:
  - Ex situ conservation and protection of important threatened plant species.
  - Serve as center of excellence for conservation, research and training.
  - Create awareness among public for conservation of plant diversity at home and outside through teaching programmes. In aid to this various zoos have been developed in country to protect endangered animal species, e.g. Manipur Thamin Deer, white-winged wood duck, white tigers, etc.
- ***Gene banks:*** The preservation of genetic material and resources is maintained through gene banks and seed banks. The National Bureau of Plant Genetic Resources (NBPGR), New Delhi has preserved seeds of wild plants, crops and cultivated varieties. The National Bureau of Animal Genetic Resource at Karnal, Haryana preserves genetic for domestic animals and genetic material of fishes is preserved by The National Bureau of Fish Genetic Resources, Lukhnow.

- ***Cryopreservation:*** This method is useful for preserving vegetative propagated crops. Cryopreservation is used to preserve meristems, zygotic and somatic embryos, pollen, protoplasts cells and suspension cultures of a number of plant species at ultra low temperature (-196°C) of liquid nitrogen.

Presently Government is taking serious action by implementing laws and rules against hunting, fishing and preservation of wild animals, fishes and various plant species for protection of natural biodiversity.

ASSESSMENT

Essay Type Questions

1. Define biodiversity. Discuss in detail about conservation of biodiversity.
2. Explain in detail about various ongoing projects of Indian Government for endangered species.
3. Discuss about facts and importance of biodiversity.

Multiple Choice Questions

1. Biodiversity is:
   (a) Variety of life on earth (b) Variety of plants on earth
   (c) Variety of animals on earth (d) Variety of ecological seasons
2. Ecological benefits of biodiversity is:
   (a) Provide food web (b) Provide fresh oxygen
   (c) Provide various medicinal plants (d) None of the above
3. The valuable species on earth are getting extinct because of:
   (a) Habitat degradation (b) Climate change
   (c) Over population (d) Ecological changes
4. Which of the following is not a site for in situ method of conservation of flora?
   (a) Biosphere reserve (b) Botanical garden
   (c) National park (d) Wildlife sanctuary

Fill in the Blanks

5. The Kanha National Park is situated in ____________.
6. The preservation of different species of both animals and plants is known as ____________.
7. The purpose to declare 'Sacred lakes and forests' is to prevent ____________ of forest animals as well as marine life.

ANSWERS

1. a	2. b	3. a	4. b
5. Madhya Pradesh	6. Conservation		7. Hunting

CHAPTER

Environmental Protection 8

Learning Objectives

At the end, students will be able to:
- Describe Environmental, Wildlife and Forest Conservation Acts.
- Describe Air and Water Pollution Acts.
- Enumerate role of NGO's in environmental protection.
- Give information on role of information technology in environmental protection and human health.

ENVIRONMENTAL PROTECTION ACT

The Environmental Protection Act was implemented on 23rd May, 1986 by Parliament of India. This act was formulated for protection and improvement of various environments and for matters connected there with.

The decision of environment act 1986 was taken at the United Nations Conference on the human environment held at Stockholm in June, 1972 in which India has participated and took efforts to implement this act.

General Powers of Central Government under Act 1986

- The central government has power of provision of this act for purpose of protecting and improving quality of environment and preventing, controlling and abating environmental pollution.
- Planning and execution of nationwide programs for the prevention control and abatement of environment pollution with support of state governments.
- Central government has authority to lay down standards for discharge of environmental pollutants from various sources, e.g. industries.
- Authority of restriction for areas of environmental pollution causing industries, operations and processes.
- Making of laws for proper handling of emissions, discharge and wastes of industries, operations and processes for environmental safeguards.
- Laying down procedures for safeguarding of environment as well as prevention of accidents.
- Laying down procedures for handling of hazardous substances and examination of materials and processes causing environmental pollution.
- Encourage experiments and research for inventions of various methods to prevent and control environmental pollution.
- Authority for inspection of premises, plants, industries, machinery and manufacturing places, etc. for carrying out recommended procedures to prevent, control and abetment of environmental pollution.

- Preparation of manuals, codes and guides relating to prevention, control and abatement of environmental pollution.
- Authority to punish any person who fails to implement the provisions of act with imprisonment for a term extending up to 5 years or penalty worth ₹ 1 Lakh or both.
- The central government is responsible to set certain laboratories in country for prevention of environmental pollution.
- The central government is also responsible for safe and effective execution of environment protection act in country.

AIR (PREVENTION AND CONTROL OF POLLUTION) ACT, INDIA

The Air (Prevention and Control of Pollution) Act was implemented by Indian government on 29th March, 1981, after planned at United Nations Conference on Human Environment held at Stockholm in 1972.

Salient Features of Act

- The Air (Prevention and Control of Pollution) Act 1981 was implemented by central and state governments.
- The sources of pollution such as industry, vehicles, power plants, etc. are not permitted to release particulate matter, lead, CO_2, SO_2, NO_2, volatile organic compounds (VOCs), etc. beyond prescribed level.
- For proper and effective implementation of this act, central government has set up pollution control boards at central and state level with the help of state governments.

Objectives of Act

- To provide prevention, control and abatement of air pollution.
- The provisions for establishment of central and state boards with a view of implementation of Act.
- To confer on the boards and powers to implement the provisions of the act and assign functions to the boards relating to Act.

Functions of Central Air Pollution Control Board

- The major function of central air pollution control board is to improve quality of air and prevention, control and abatement of air pollution.
- Central board coordinate with central government to give advice on any matter concerning of air pollution control and prevention to improve quality of air.
- Central board plan and execute the nationwide air pollution prevention, control and abatement programs.
- Coordinate activities of state boards and is responsible to dissolve disputes among them.
- Central board provides technical assistance and guidance to state boards to implement research procedures for invention of methods to prevent, control and abatement of air pollution.
- Plan and execute training programs for workers engaged in prevention, control and abatement of air pollution programs.

- Organize a comprehensive program through mass media regarding air pollution and control.
- Lay down standards for quality of air as well as collect and disseminate information of matters regarding air pollution prevention and control programs and Act.
- Delegate the work and duties to appointed committees to control air pollution.

Functions of State Board

- To plan and secure execution of a comprehensive program for prevention, control and abatement of air pollution.
- To advise state government on any matter related to prevention, control and abatement of air pollution.
- To collect and disseminate information regarding various air pollution control programs and Act.
- To collaborate with central board for organization of training program for workers engaged in air pollution prevention and control programs.
- To inspect periodically any control equipment, industrial plant or manufacturing process at risk to produce air pollutants.
- To inspect and investigate air pollution control areas and programs time-to-time to assess quality of work and needed improvement.
- To lay down standards of air pollution prevention, control and abatement with coordination of central board and is highly responsible for effective execution of these standards in required areas.
- To advise state government with respect to the suitability of any premises or location for carrying on any industry this is likely to cause air pollution.
- A state board must establish laboratories to function under this section efficiently regarding air pollution.
- To collect, complete and publish statistical census regarding air pollution with coordination of state government.

■ WATER (PREVENTION AND CONTROL OF POLLUTION) ACT

The Water (Prevention and Control of Pollution) Act was implemented on 23rd March, 1974 and was amended in 1988. This act was established by central government with association of boards at central and state level for prevention and control of water pollution.

Water Pollution Cess Act

This act was established in 1977 and was amended in 2003. The objective of this act was to impose cess rate on consumption of water by any type and level on consumer.

Objectives of Act

The act was formulated for purpose of prevention and control of water pollution and the maintenance and restoration of wholesome water.

Functions of Central Water Pollution Control Board

- To advise the central government on any matter concerning the prevention and control of water pollution.

- To coordinate the activities of the state boards and resolve disputes among them.
- The major function is to provide technical assistance and guidance to the state boards, carry out and sponsor investigations and research relating to problems of water pollution and prevention, control or abatement of water pollution.
- To plan and organize the training of persons engaged or to be engaged in programs for the prevention, control or abatement of water pollution.
- To organize a comprehensive program through mass media regarding the prevention and control of water pollution.
- To collect, compile and publish technical and statistical data relating to water pollution and the measures devised for its effective prevention and control and prepare manuals, codes or guides relating to treatment and disposal of sewage and trade effluents and disseminate information connected therewith.
- To lay down, modify or annul, in consultation with the state government concerned, the standards for a stream or well.
- To plan and execute a nationwide program for the prevention, control or abatement of water pollution.

Functions of State Water Pollution Control Board

- To plan a comprehensive program for the prevention, control or abatement of pollution of streams and wells in the state and to secure the execution of these programs.
- To advise the state government on any matter concerning the prevention, control or abatement of water pollution.
- To collect and disseminate information relating to water pollution and the prevention control or abatement of water pollution.
- To encourage, conduct and participate in investigations and research relating to problems of water pollution and prevention, control or abatement of water pollution.
- To collaborate with the central board in organizing the training of persons engaged or to be engaged in programs relating to prevention, control or abatement of water pollution and to organize mass education programs relating these programs.
- To inspect sewage or trade effluents, works and plants for the treatment of sewage and trade effluents and to review plans, specifications or other data relating to plants set up for the treatment of water, works for the purification of water and the system for the disposal of sewage.
- To lie down, modify annul effluent standards for the sewage and trade effluents and for the quality of receiving waters (not being water in an interstate stream) resulting from the discharge of effluents.
- To collect, compile and publish technical and statistical data relating to water pollution and the measured devices for its effective prevention and control as well as to prepare manuals, codes or guides relating to treatment and disposal of sewage and trade effluents and disseminate information connected with them.

- To lie down and modify standards in consultation with the state government concerned with a stream or well by means of types of source, quality of water flow characteristics, etc.
- To plan and execute a nationwide program for the prevention, control or abatement of water pollution.
- The board must establish or recognize a laboratory or laboratories to enable the board to perform its functions under this section efficiently, including the analysis of samples of water from any stream or well or of samples of any sewage or trade effluents.

The Wildlife (Protection) Act

The Wildlife (Protection) Act was executed on 9th September, 1972 by Parliament of India and was amended in 1993, 2002 and 2006. The recent amendments were passed by Rajya Sabha on 64th republic day of nation in 2013.

Objectives of Act

- To provide protection to wild animals, birds and plants for conservation of biodiversity of nation.
- To protect and implement procedures to prevent hunting and accidents to wildlife.
- To deal with matters related to wildlife.

Salient Features of Wildlife Act

- The act contains 66 sections with 7 chapters and 6 schedules.
- ***Chapter I:*** This chapter includes preliminary features of an act:
  - The act is extends to whole of India except state Jammu and Kashmir.
  - This act will be enforced into state and union territories on same date of bill, i.e. 9th September, 1972.
- ***Chapter II:*** This chapter includes appointment of authorities for conservation of wildlife. The central government is responsible to appoint:
  - ***Appointment of directors and officers***
    - Director of wildlife preservation
    - Assistant directors of wildlife preservation
    - Other officers and employees as may be necessary.
  - ***Appointment of chief wildlife warden and other officers***
    - Chief wildlife warden
    - Wildlife wardens (one honorary wildlife warden in each district)
    - Other officers.
  - ***Power of delegation***
    - The director has authority to delegate the duties to subordinates with approval of central government.
    - The chief wildlife warden has authority to delegate duties to subordinates with approval of state government.
  - ***Constitution of wildlife advisory board:*** The wildlife advisory board of any state and union territory will be constituted of
    - The incharge minister of forest department (alternative is chief secretary to state government) will be chairman of board

- Two members of state legislature
- Secretary to state government incharge of forest department
- Incharge forest officer of state
- An officer nominated by director
- Chief wildlife warden
- Other forest department officers of state
- Other persons.

■ ***Functions of wildlife advisory board:*** The wildlife advisory board has to advise the state government regarding:
- The selection of areas to be declared as sanctuaries, national parks, and closed areas.
- In formulation of the policy of protection and conservation of wildlife and specified plants.
- In any matter relating to any schedule of Wildlife Act.
- In relation to the measures to be taken for harmonizing the needs of the tribal and other dwellers of the forest with the protection and conservation of wildlife.
- In any matter that may be referred to it by the state government.

- ***Chapter III:*** This chapter is related to hunting of wild animals and protection of wild plants:
  - No person shall hunt any wild animal
  - ***Permission of hunting wild animals in certain cases as following:***
    - The chief wildlife can permit to hunt any wild animal if he become dangerous for human life, disabled, diseased and is beyond recovery.
    - The killing or wounding of any wild animal is permit able in self defense and in saving to other person but the dead body of animal will be property of government.
    - Hunting is allowed for special purposes like education, scientific research, scientific management, collection of specimens (for zoos and museums).
    - The chief wildlife has authority to cancel license for hunting in any condition with generous reason.
  - ***Protection for plants***
    - The picking, uprooting, etc. of specified wild plants is prohibited.
    - The willful pick, sale, destroy, damage, transfer uprooting of any wild plant without permission of central government is offense able.
    - Permission for picking and uprooting of wild plant is in certain conditions like education, scientific research, collection, preservation and display in scientific institution.
- ***Chapter IV:*** This chapter involves matter related to declaration of sanctuaries, national parks and closed areas:
  - ***Declaration of national parks:*** The state government declares any area other than comprised with any reserve forest or territorial water as sanctuary.
  - ***Declaration of national parks:*** The state government declares the area as national park by reason of its ecological, faunal, floral, geomorphologic and zoological importance.

- **Declaration of closed area:** The state government declares to any area prohibited for hunting to prevent wildlife.

- ***Chapter V:*** This chapter deals with central zoo authority and recognition of zoos:
  - The central government constitute a central zoo authority comprised of
    - A chairperson
    - Ten members
    - Members (secretary to be appointed by central government).
  - Functions of central zoo authority
    - Specify the minimum standards for housing, unkeep and veterinary care of the animals kept in a zoo.
    - Evaluate and assess the functioning of zoos with respect to the standards or the norms as may be prescribed recognized or derecognized of zoo.
    - Identify endangered species of wild animals for purposes of captive breeding and assigning responsibility in this regard to a zoo.
    - Coordinate the acquisition, exchange and loaning of animals for breeding purposes.
    - Ensure maintenance of studbooks of endangered species of wild animals bred in captivity.
    - Identify priorities and themes with regard to display of captive animals in a zoo.
    - Coordinate training of zoo personnel in India and outside India.
- ***Chapter VI:*** This chapter involves trades or commerce in wild animals, animal articles and trophies.
  - The wild animals killed by mistake, during defense, found dead will be government's property.
  - The writing and publication of any specific wild animal without permission of central government and chief wildlife will be punishable and declare as government's property.
  - The trades of animal trophies and manufacturing of trophies made up of animal parts is declared as punishable offense and will be government's property.
- ***Chapter VII:*** This chapter is related to prevention and detection of offences.
  - ***Power of entry, search, arrest and detention:*** Any forest department employee authorized by director on the behalf of chief wildlife can:
    - Inspect any person for captive animal, wild animal, meat and animal article and can take him in his custody, take possession of license, any document, etc.
    - Stop any vehicle for search on the basis of suspiciousness of captive animal, wild animal, etc.
  - ***Penalties:***
    - Any person who found to breach the rules of license or permit granted under this act can be imprisoned for a term extending up to 3 years or fine up to ₹ 25,000 or both.

- A person found guilty to commit offence in relation to wild animal, meat, animal trophy or an animal article in forest, national park or sanctuary will be punished with imprisonment of a term not less than one year extending up to six year and fine up to ₹ 5000.

THE FOREST (CONSERVATION) ACT

The act was provided for conservation of forests and for matters related to the natural habitat of flora and fauna. The act was enforced on 25th October, 1980 and amendments were done in 1988 by parliamentary constitution of India.

Salient Features of Act

- Restriction is there on use of land of reserved forests and use for a forestation is offence able.
- The use of forest land for nonforest purposes such as cultivation of tea, coffee, rubber, horticulture of medicinal plants, etc. is a crime and punishable.
- Clearance of any forest land of naturally grown trees for the purpose of reforestation is forbidden.

ROLE OF NGO'S IN ENVIRONMENTAL EDUCATION/ ENVIRONMENTAL PROTECTION

Today we came across various nongovernmental organizations (NGO) working in different areas of country for betterment of society as well as nation and to bring positive change among people. They contribute a lot in development of country by working on various missions like women welfare, orphans welfare, environmental protection, etc.

Definition: A NGO is any nonprofit voluntary citizen's group which is organized on a local, national and international level, task-oriented and driven by people with a common interest.

Role of NGO's in Environmental Education and Protection

- ***General functions***
  - Evoke consciousness regarding surrounding environment among people by acting as catalyst.
  - Make awareness and implementation of proper enactment of legislation
  - Working on self help basis.
  - Articulate interests of vulnerable and neglected parts of environment protection.
- ***Role of NGO's in protection of environment:***
  - They create public awareness regarding burning issues of environment and solutions to those issues.
  - Facilitates the participation of various categories of stakeholders in discussion on environmental issues.
  - Create awareness for protection of human rights for clean environments as well as duties towards safe environment.
  - Help in protecting natural resources and entrusting the equitable use of resources.

- Generate recent data on natural resources.
- Analyze and monitor the environmental quality .
- Helps the rural administration in preparation, application and execution of proposals on environmental protection.
- Help in disseminate information through mass media, internet, articles and AV aids, etc.
- Organize seminars, conferences, dramas, discussions for awareness of environmental protection.

ROLE OF INFORMATION TECHNOLOGY IN ENVIRONMENT AND HUMAN HEALTH

Role of Information Technology in Environment

The important roles of information technology in environment are as follows:

- ***Database:*** Database involves the collection of interrelated data on various subjects and is usually in computerized that can be retrieved whenever required. The different distribution information centers of nation are interrelated to each other as well as to globe through database. The government of India has taken up project of compiling data on various issues like wildlife, forest cover, wastelands, etc.
- ***Environmental Information System (ENVIS):*** ENVIS work to generate a network for database in various areas like pollution control, clean technologies, biodiversity, renewable energy, wildlife, etc. and help in providing information to policy makers, scientists and engineer.

  Objectives of ENVIS
  - To build up a repository and dissemination center in environmental science and engineering.
  - To gear up modern technologies of acquiring, processing, storage, retrieval and dissemination of information of environmental nature.
  - To promote research, development and innovation in environmental information technology.
  - To provide national environmental information service relevant to meet the future needs.

  ENVIS network: ENVIS provides a huge network of various institutes participating in forming a number of nodes called ENVIS centers those work with a focal point in the Ministry of Environment and Forest, thus ENVIS is known as National Focal Point (NFP) for INFOTERRA, a global environmental information network of United Nations Environment Programme (UNEP).
- ***Remote sensing:*** Remote sensing technique through satellite can be used to assess ongoing changes in the environment and to predict natural calamities like droughts, floods and volcanic eruptions, etc. The technique is of great use in exploring the possible availability of crude oils, mineral deposits and location of geothermal power sources.
- ***National Management Information System (NMIS):*** NMIS of the department of science and technology has compiled a database on research and

development projects along with information about research scientists and personnel involved.

- ***Geographical Information System (GIS):*** GIS is a technique of superimposing various thematic maps using digital data on a large number of interrelated or interdependent aspects like water resources, forest land, soil type, crop land, industrial growth, human settlement, etc. are superimposed in a layered form in computer using softwares.

  Applications of GIS: GIS can be used in:
  - Prospective land use planning, interpretation of polluted zones and degraded lands.
  - Providing information of atmospheric phenomenon like approach of monsoon, ozone layer depletion, smog and inversion phenomenon, etc.
  - Planning for locating suitable areas for industrial growth.
  - Play a key role in resource mapping, environmental conservation and environmental impact assessment.

Role of Information Technology in Human Health

Information technology is playing a major role in various areas related to human health like:

- Bioinformatics
- Genome sequencing
- Gene engineering
- Online medical transcription
- Telemedicine
- Database used for maintenance of human health
- Biotechnology
- Identification of several diseases, infected areas and areas prone to vector born disease, e.g malaria, schistosomiasis, etc.

ASSESSMENT

Essay Type Questions

1. Define Environmental Protection Act and explain in detail about its salient features.
2. Give in detail about role of NGO's in environmental education and protection.

Short Answer Type Questions

1. Define database.
2. Enlist objectives of Air (Protection and Control of Pollution) Act.
3. Describe in brief about Environmental Information System (ENVIS).

Multiple Choice Questions

1. The Water Pollution Cess Act was launched in year of:
   (a) 1988 (b) 1980
   (c) 1977 (d) 1981
2. The United Nations conference on environment was held at Stockholm in year of:
   (a) 1982 (b) 1992
   (c) 2002 (d) 1972
3. The Wildlife (Protection) Act was recently amended in year of:
   (a) 2013 (b) 2014
   (c) 2015 (d) 2016
4. As per chapter II of the Wildlife (Protection) Act, the authority to delegation of duties hold:
   (a) The chief wildlife warden (b) The warden
   (c) The director (d) The assistant director
5. The area possessing specific ecological. Faunal and floral importance is declared as:
   (a) Sanctuary (b) Closed area
   (c) National park (d) None of the above

ANSWERS

1. c 2. d 3. a 4. c
5. c

CHAPTER

9 Disaster Management

Learning Objectives

At the end of unit, students will be able to:
- Define disaster.
- Describe types of disaster.
- Define disaster management.
- Describe phases of disaster management.

DISASTER

Introduction

The event suddenly that happen causing mass harm to life, economics and natural environment can be disaster. Disasters can be in any form like droughts, floods, volcanoes, storms, tsunamis etc. with different level of frequency, duration and destruction. The word disaster coined form French term 'desastre' and Italian 'disastro' that means bad star.

Definition

A disaster is a serious disruption, occurring over a relatively short time, of the functioning of a community or a society involving widespread human, material, economic or environmental loss and impacts, which exceeds the ability of the affected community or society to cope using its own resources.

Or

A sudden calamitous event bringing great damage, loss, or destruction natural disasters; broadly: a sudden or great misfortune or failure.

Or

The Disaster Management Act 2005 defines a disaster as 'a catastrophes mishap, calamity or grave occurrence from natural and manmade causes, which is beyond the coping capacity of the affected community.

Types of Disasters

The disasters can be classified into two types based on their form of occurrence as follows:
- ***Natural disasters:*** This involves the natural occurring of physical phenomena caused either by rapid or slow onset of events related to geophysical, hydrological, climatologically, meteorological or biological. The examples for this are floods, droughts, diseases, earthquakes, cyclones etc.

- ***Man-made disasters:*** These are also known as technological disasters. These are the events occur due to human activities causing environmental degradation, pollution and accidents. The example for this is nuclear blast, explosions, industrial accidents, etc.

Phases of Disasters

The disaster has three phases:
1. Pre-impact phase
2. Impact phase
3. Post impact.

DISASTER MANAGEMENT

Definition

Disaster management can be defined as the organization and management of resources and responsibilities for dealing with all humanitarian aspects of emergencies, in particular preparedness, response and recovery in order to lessen the impact of disasters.

Aims of Disaster Management

- To reduce damages and deaths.
- To reduce personal sufferings of victims.
- To enhance the speed of recovery.
- To protect victims from further damage.

Principles of Disaster Management

- Disaster management is the responsibility of all spheres of government.
- Disaster management should use resources that exist for a day-to-day purpose.
- Organizations should function as an extension of their core business.
- Individuals are responsible for their own safety.
- Disaster management planning should focus on large-scale events.

Phases of Disaster Management

Disaster management consists of following phases:
- Disaster prevention
- Disaster preparedness
- Disaster impact and response
- Recovery and rehabilitation
- Disaster mitigation.

Prevention

- Prevention includes the activities those are designed for permanent protection from disaster.
- The risk of injury and life can be minimized with good plan of early evacuation, environmental planning and design standards.
- In January 2005, 168 countries adopted a 10-year global plan known as The Hyogo Framework for natural disaster risk and that includes guiding

principles, priorities for action and practical means for achieving disaster resilience for vulnerable communities.

Disaster Preparedness

Preparedness is focused on preparing equipments and procedures for use when a disaster occurs.

Preparedness should not be in form of money and manpower but as follows:

- This is ongoing multisectoral activity.
- This is a long-term goal of country to strengthen the overall capacity and capability to manage any sort of emergency arrived.
- This preparation can be done by the critique assessment of previous experiences of disasters in country.
- The detection of disaster prone areas.
- Adopt standards and regulations at the place of risk.
- Organize communication, information and instillation of warning system and devices.
- Ensure coordination and response mechanism.
- Develop public education and training program.
- Coordinate with media for information sessions.
- Organize disaster simulation exercise that test response mechanism.
- Keep stocks of food, drugs and other essential commodities.
- The United Nation Agencies those provide humanitarian assistance are UNICEF, WHO, International Committee of Red Cross, CARE etc.

Disaster Impact and Response

Disaster impact is the result of occurrence of disaster and most injuries sustained during impact. Thus first few hours after disaster are very crucial and need immediate action.

The management during this time period can be as follows:

- ***Search, rescue and first aid:***
  - After a major disaster, the first action needed is searching and rescue of non injured and less injured people from disaster place.
  - These less injured people can help in rescue of other victims after first aid management.
- ***Field care:***
  - The rescue team should divide people in small groups for different rescue works and choose one leader who will direct rescue work and will keep documentation.
  - Major injured people need immediate medical care thus; first priority is to inform medical team about disaster and place.
  - Transport victims to near medical facility center with any available transport medium.
  - Inform nearby hospitals to increase bed availability and to keep ready for surgical interventions.
  - Establish a center very near at safe place to respond to inquiries from relatives of victims and try to collect maximum information regarding

victims, i.e. numbers of victims for particular type of injury, number of deaths, names of victims, etc.

- Priority should be given to victim's identification.
- Space should be prepared near to disaster place for using as mortuary for dead victims.
- Provisions for food and shelter should be made for survivors.

- ***Triage:***
  - When severity of impact and quantity of victims increased medical team can follow a new approach.
  - The principal of ' First come first treated ' is not be followed during mass emergency and Triage can be followed.
  - The triage is division of victims into groups on the basis of severity of injuries and chances of survival.
  - The priority for emergency care should be given to victims with less injury and high chances of survival.
  - The international triage system followed four color codes.
  - ***Green color:*** Victims need immediate attention because of less injury and are ambulatory. The chances of survival for these victims are high and are not in need of transfer to hospital. For example victims with laceration, minor injuries, etc.
  - ***Yellow color:*** The victims of second priority who may or may not ambulate but has high survival rate and need transfer to hospital but these patients can wait for exact treatment. The victims having injuries like minor fractures, fractures of limbs, minor muscle injuries, etc.
  - ***Red color:*** The victims with life-threatening injuries, unconscious and need immediate transfer to hospital for emergency care and surgical interventions. These victims have less or no chances of survival. For example people with head injuries, blunt traumas, multiple injuries, etc.
  - ***Black color:*** This color code is used for dead or moribund victims.
- ***Tagging:*** All victims should be identified with tags stating their name, age, place of origin, triage category, diagnosis and initial treatment.
- ***Identification of dead:*** A large number of dead can interrupt the rescue activity at the site of disaster thus care of dead need attention as follows:
  - Removal of dead from the disaster scene
  - Shifting to the mortuary
  - Identification of dead
  - Reception of bereaved relatives
  - Legal procedure of handing over the body.
- ***Relief phase:***
  - This phase begins after immediate rescue and triage process when outer assistance arrived.
  - The supplies of health care are needed immediately after emergency phase which can be measured as local availability and effect of distinct events on population.
  - Initial phase includes supply of medical care needs followed by food and clothing, shelter, sanitary engineering equipment and construction material.

  - The four principles can be followed for humanitarian assistance after receiving donations: 1. acquisition of supplies, 2. transportation, 3. storage and 4. distribution.
- Epidemiological surveillance:
  - The risk of epidemiological disease outbreak increase at disaster and rescue site because of overcrowding, poor sanitation, damage to local water resources and sewage system, etc.
  - The prevention of disease should be done with:
    - Implementation of public health measures as soon as possible.
    - Organize a reliable disease reporting system.
    - Identify at initial of disease outbreak and control measures.
    - Investigate all reports of disease outbreak rapidly.
    - Vaccination for contagious disease should be making available through cold chain system.
- ***Nutrition:*** Due to disastrous conditions the scarcity of food occur leading to nutritional problems among people. The risk prone victims like children, pregnant women, nursing mothers can suffer from malnutrition. Thus:
  - Assess food supply after disaster.
  - Gauge the nutritional needs of affected population.
  - Calculate daily food rations and need for large population groups.
  - Monitoring the nutritional status of affected population.

Rehabilitation

This is final phase in disaster that leads to restoration of pre-disaster conditions.

Rehabilitation starts from very first moment of disaster. It includes:

- Reestablishment of pre disaster and normal conditions.
- Reorganization and restructure of services needed.
- The safe water supply to area should be restored.
- Ensure excreta disposal in proper manner to prevent disease outbreak.
- Proper disposal method of sewage and waste disposal should be reestablished.
- Personal hygiene maintenance should be encouraged and facilities should be provided.
- Safe food restoration should be enhanced.
- Vector control programs should be launched as soon as possible.

Phase of Mitigation

This phase involves lessening the effects of disaster.

- Protecting vulnerable population and structure like.
- By improving structural qualities of school, providing general health care system, etc.
- By ensuring public health services like safe water supply, sanitation facilities, etc.

Disaster Recovery

- Successful recovery preparation
- Be vigilant in health teaching

- Psychological support
- Referrals to hospital as needed
- Remain alert for environmental health.

Major Disasters of India

- 1984 Bhopal gas tragedy
- 2001 Gujarat earthquake
- 2004 Indian ocean tsunami
- 2008 Mumbai attacks
- 2013 Uttarakhand floods and landslides
- 2013 floods in Assam.

Disaster Management Act in India

India is one of the 10th disaster prone countries of the world and losing about 2% GDP on its disasters. It is highly vulnerable to floods, droughts, forest fires, cyclones, landslides and earthquakes. Out of total 36 states and union territory, 28 out of them are disaster prone.

National Policy on Disaster Management 2009

The policy aims at developing an integrated , holistic, multidisaster oriented and technology driven strategy for disaster management involving, mitigation, preparedness, response and prevention at various level (national, state and district).

Disaster Management Act of India

The Disaster Management Act was executed on 23rd December, 2005 by constitution of India.

Salient Features of Disaster Management

- The prime minister of country would be chairperson of committee.
- The chairperson will nominate nine members of committee.
- The committee members will act as coordinating and monitoring body of disaster management team.
- The committee will prepare national plan with help of national authority of disaster management.
- The committee will lie down guidelines for disaster management plan and will monitor the implementation of guidelines and policies at disaster site.
- The committee will provide technical assistance and guidance to disaster management team.
- The committee will plan for training and simulation of various disasters management teams.
- The committee will recommend provision for funds for mitigation and rehabilitation.

ASSESSMENT

Essay Type Questions

1. Define disaster. Discuss about types of disaster.
2. Define disaster management. Explain in detail about disaster management.

Multiple Choice Questions

1. The sudden climates loss and destruction is called:
   (a) Disaster (b) Deforestation
   (c) Weather change d) Soil erosion
2. The earthquake is an example of:
   (a) Man-made disaster (b) Natural disaster
   (c) Both (a) and (b) (d) None of the above
3. The example of man-made disaster is:
   (a) Drought (b) Hurricane
   (c) Deforestation (d) Nuclear explosion
4. The distribution of disaster victims as per color coding is process of:
   (a) Rescue (b) Rehabilitation
   (c) Triage (d) Mitigation
5. The color code used for dead victims of disaster is:
   (a) Green (b) Red
   (c) Yellow (d) Black

ANSWERS

1. (a) 2. (b) 3. (d) 4. (c)
5. (d)

Index

Page numbers followed by *f* refer to figure and *t* refer to table.

A

Abortion 42
Accidental spills and leaks 44
Acid rain 14, 95, 96
  causes of 95
  formation of 96
  solution of 97
  types of 95
Acidity, higher 47
Activated sludge process 68
  procedure of 68
Activated sludge system 69*f*
Adaptations 102
Aerobic composting 62
  types of 62*f*
Aerobic process 66
Agricultural machines 41
Agriculture 91
  on food resources, adverse impact of 16
  pollutants 44
Air 36, 37, 108
  chemical composition of 37
  conditioning 52
  flow, sudden change in direction of 39
  physical properties of 37
  pollutants and effects 38
  pollution 36, 37, 39
    control measures of 38
    sources of 37
    technical methods to control 39
  standard component of 37
Airborne disease 40
  uncommon 40
Alkaline pH 26
Aluminium recycling 61
Amebiasis 31
Anaerobic
  digestion 63
  process 66
Anthrax 40
Anti-oxidant 26
Aquatic
  biomes 71
  ecosystem 85
    types of 85
  host 31
Atmosphere 5
Atmospheric air, properties of normal 37
Atmospheric contaminants 28
Automobile sources 37
Autotrophs 74

B

Bacillary dysentery 31
Back washing 36
Balanced ventilation 52
Basic needs 12
Bathing and washing 51
Bed of graded sand 34
Bin/pile composting 62
Biodiversity 101, 102
  conservation 103
  division of 101
  hotspots of 102
  in situ conservation of 104
  levels of 101
Biogeochemistry 77
Biological
  environment 4
  magnification 17
  pollutants 44
  treatment plant 64
  water treatment plant 65*f*
Biomass 18, 74

Biomedical waste 58
 management 58, 59, 59*f*
 types of 58*f*
Biosphere 5, 71
 reserves 104
Biotic components 73, 73*t*
Biotic environment 4
Birth rate 90, 91
Black carbon 97
Bleaching powder 31, 33
Blood pressure, ratings of 42
Boiling 31
Botanical garden 105

C

Canopy 83
Carbon
 cycle 79, 79*f*
 monoxide 38
Carnivores 74
Catchment 23
Central air pollution control board, functions of 108
Central Government under Act, general powers of 107
Central water pollution control board, functions of 109
Charcoal filter 23, 23*f*
Chemical 30
 disinfection 31
 salts 28
 waste 58
  dumping 44
Chemosynthesis 74
Child mortality rate 90
Chloride content 25
Chlorinated lime 31
Chlorine solution 32
Chlorofluorocarbons 99
Choking marine life 47
Cholera 31
Climate change 14, 17, 97, 98, 103
 causes of 97
Climatic conditions 88
Coagulation 35
Coal 15, 18
 ash 48
Cold desert 85
Combustion 39
Commercial chemical products waste 58
Common airborne diseases 40
Common cold 40
Communication 88
Community
 and homes 9
 ecosystem 73
 role 43
Components, abiotic 73, 73*t*
Composting bin/pile 62*f*
Concentration, lack of 42
Coniferous forests 82
Conserve water, easy steps to 29
Constitution of Wildlife Advisory Board 111
Consumers 4, 74
Contaminant free 26
Control measures 92
Controlling gaseous pollutants, methods of 39
Controlling particulate emissions, methods of 39
Crocodile breeding and management project 105
Croplands 16
Crude birth rate 89
Crude death rate 90
Crude oil 15
Cryogenic processes 97
Cryopreservation 106
Cryptosporidium 31
Current environmental issues 88
Cyclops 31

D

Dams 14
Dead, identification of 121
Death rate 91
Declaration of closed area 113
Declining population 89
Decomposers 5, 75
Defense trainings 41
Deforestation 13, 92
Delegation, power of 111
Deritivores 75
Desert ecosystem 85
 types of 85
Detergents 58
Diarrhea 30, 31
Diffusion 52
Diphtheria 40

Disaster 118
  impact and response 120
  major 123
  management 118, 119, 123
    aims of 119
    phases of 119
    principles of 119
  man-made 119
  phases of 119
  preparedness 120
  recovery 122
  types of 118
Diseases, control of 91
Domestic sources 38
Double pot method 33
Drainage system 34
Droughts 14
Dry deciduous forests 83
Dry deposition 95
Dry phase 85
Dysentery 30

E

E. coli 31
Earth
  components of 6
  layers of 7*f*
  water supply, distribution of 6*f*
Eastern Himalaya's biodiversity 102
Ecological
  diversity 101
  services 102
  succession 77
  system, energy in 75
Ecology 71, 72
  levels of 71
Economy 91, 102
Ecosystem 14, 71, 72
  biotic components of 74, 74*f*
  components of 73, 73*f*
  concept of 72
  functions of 75
  process of 75
  structure of 75, 76*f*
  types of 82
Electrostatic precipitators 39
Energy
  flow 77
  recovery 63
  resources 17
    consumption of 15

Environment 1, 7
  composition of 4
  hazard 92
  population explosion of 92
  types of 4
Environmental
  engineering 3
  health 8, 9
  hygiene 1
  information system 115
  management 3
  pollution 21
  protection Act 107
  science 2–4
    principles of 2
    scope and importance of 3
  studies and environmental pollution
      control 3
Epidemiological surveillance 122
Equator 6
Eutrophication 17
Evapotranspiration 78
Ex situ conservation 104, 105
Exhaust ventilation 52
Exosphere 6
Extreme weather patterns 100

F

Fabric filters 39
Family planning facilities 93
Fatigue 42
Fertility ratio 90
Fertilizers related problems 17
Field care 120
Filter 23
  beds 35
  box 34
  cleaning 35
  control 35
    valves, system of 34
Filtration 34, 36
  biological method of 34
  of water 32
First flush 23
Fish tape worm 31
Fisheries 16
Flocculation 35
Floods 16
Floor 50
  area 51

Food 13, 14
- and drink 12
- chain 77, 78*f*
  - trophic level 77*f*
- production resources, types of 16
- resources 15
  - problems with 16
- variety of 102
- web 76

Forest (conservation) Act 114
Forest
- ecosystem 82
  - functions of 84
- floor 83
- resources 13
- structure of 83

Fossil fuels 18
Foundry activities 44
Fresh water availability 92
Fuel minerals 15

G

Garbage and refuse 51
Gene banks 105
General health effects 42
Genetic diversity 101
Geographical ecosystem 72
Geographical information system 116
Geological disposal 49
Geothermal energy 18
Giardia 31
Giardiasis 31
Glass material recycling 61
Global changes 17
Global dimming 100
Global warming 17, 92, 99, 100
Government's role 42
Grassland
- ecosystem 84
- functions of 84
- structure of 84
- types of 84

Gravity 39
Greenhouse gases 97
Grit chamber 67
Ground level ozone 38
Groundwater 78
- pollution 28

Growth, basis of 89
Guinea worm 31

H

Habitat 14
- degradation/loss 103
- protection of 104

Hard water 24
Hazardous wastes 9
Hazards of mining 15
Health 7
- ill effects on 37

Healthy environment, importance of 7, 8
Healthy house, construction of 50
Healthy housing 50
Helminthic 31
Hepatitis
- A 31
- E 31

Herbaceous layer 83
Herbivores 74
Heterotrophs 74
Hot desert 85
Household 41
- methods for purification of water 31

Housing 49
- aims of 49
- and infrastructures 12
- and ventilation 49
- location of 50
- site of 50
- standards 50

Human activities 44
Human health 96
- and urbanization 93
- dangers to 47
- impacts of poor housing on 51

Human population and environment 88
Humidity 37
Hydatid disease 31
Hydrocarbons 57
Hydrologic cycle 78, 79*f*
Hydropower 14
Hydrosphere 6
Hygienic conditions, proper 44
Hypochlorite, high test 32

I

Ice desert 85
In situ conservation 104
Industrial sources 41

Industrial waste 44, 58
Industrialization 92
Industrialized agricultural food resources 16
Infant
  mortality rate 90, 91
    lowering 93
Infective agent 31*t*
Influenza 40
Information technology in
  environment, role of 115
  human health, role of 116
Inorganic renewable 12
Insecticides 57
Intestinal worms 30
Iodine 32

K

Kitchen 51

L

Lake ecosystem 86
Land
  biomes 71
  degradation 16
Landfills 28, 44
Late marriage 92
Lead 38
Legislation 93
Leptospiral 31
Lighting 51
Literacy level 93
Lithosphere 6
Living things 96

M

Macroenvironment 4
Marine
  biodiversity 101
  ecosystem 86
  energy 19
  life, effects on 42
  pollution 45
    control measures of 47
    effects of 45, 46
    sources of 45
Material cycling in ecosystem 77
Material, recycling of 60*f*
Measles 40
Mechanical devices 39
Mechanical ventilation 52
Medicines 13
Meningitis 40
Mesosphere 6
Metallic 12
  minerals 15
Micro-clustered 26
Microenvironment 4
Micronutrient imbalance 17
Mineral
  resources 14, 15
  rich 26
Mining 13
Mitigation, phase of 122
Mobility 12
Modern agriculture on food resources, effects of 17
Moist deciduous forests 83
Mortality rate, under 5 90
Mumps 40
Municipal solid waste 59
Municipal waste 57

N

National green tribunal Act 98
National management information system 115
National mission for
  green 98
  strategic knowledge for climate change 98
  sustainable agriculture 98
  sustaining Himalayan ecosystem 98
National mission on sustainable habitat 98
National parks and sanctuaries 104
National Policy on Disaster Management 2009 123
National Solar Mission 98
National Water Mission 98
Natural
  accumulation 43
  disasters 118
  fertilizers, production of 45
  gas 15, 18
  pollutants 43
  production 44
  resources 11, 13, 38
    importance of 12
    of forests, problems with 13
    types of 11
  ventilation 52

NGOs in environmental education and protection, role of 114
Nitrate pollution 17
Nitrogen
content 25
cycle 80, 81*f*
dioxide 38
source 5
Noise 41
pollution 41
effects of 42
preventive measures for 42
sources of 41
Non-industrial sources 41
Non-living things 96
Non-metallic
minerals 15
Non-point sources 27
Non-renewable resources 12, 18
types of 12
Non-specific source waste 58
Non-standard component 37
Nuclear
energy 19
power plants 48
weapons
decomposition of 48
production of 48
Nutrient pollution 27
Nutrition 122

O

Ocean acidification 100
Ocean energy 19
Off-site conservation 104, 105
Omnivores 74
Organic
matter, decomposition of 66
renewable 12
waste, types of 57
Organisms 73
death of useful 17
Oscillating wave surge converter 19
Outdoor air quality 9
Overgrazing 16
Oxygen
cycle 80, 80*f*
depletion 46
Ozone depletion 98, 99

P

Packaging items, avoidance of 45
Paper 13
recycling 60
process of 61
Paratyphoid fever 31
Particulate matter 38
Penalties 113
Per capita income 92
Permanent deafness 42
Pertusis 40
Pesticide related problems 17
Petroleum 15
and oil 18
Phosphorus cycle 81, 81*f*
Photosynthesis 5, 74
Physical components 5
Physical environment 4
Physical treatment plant 64
Plants, protection for 112
Plenum ventilation 52
Point absorber 19
Poliomyelitis 31
Pollutants, man-made 44
Pollution 92, 103
prevention and control of 108
Polychlorinated biphenyl 57
Pond ecosystem 85
Population 73
distribution of 88
explosion 90, 91
globally, causes of 90
factors affecting distribution of 88
growth 89
measure 89
over 91
types of 44, 89
Potassium permanganate 32
Poverty 91
Power of entry 113
Primary consumers 74
Primary sedimentation 67
Primary treatment 66
Prime Minister's National Action Plan for climate changes 98
Privacy 51
Producers 74
Programs and legislation related to water cleanliness 36
Project elephant 105
Project tiger 105

Protective blanket 5
Protozoal 31
Psychological environment 4
Public address system 41
Public awareness about environment 7
PVC pipe filter 24, 24*f*

R

Radioactive
  pollutants 44, 47
  pollution 48
    causes of 48
    effects of 48
    sources of 48
  waste
    prevention and management 49
    re-use of 49
Radioactivity 47
Rainwater 22
  harvesting 22
Rangelands 16
Rapid depletion of high grade minerals 15
Rapid mixing 35
Rapid sand filter 35
  steps of process by 35
Rapidly growing population 89
Raw material 11
Refuse derived fuel 63
Regional changes 17
Rehabilitation 122
Relationship within ecosystem 72*f*
Relief phase 121
Religious belief 91
Remote sensing 115
Renewable resources 11, 18
River ecosystem 86
Road salts 28
Rooftop rainwater harvesting 23
Rotavirus diarrhea 31
Roundworm 31

S

Sacred forests 105
Sacred lakes 105
Safe drinking water, characteristics of 26
Salinity problems 17
Sand gravel filter 23, 23*f*
Sanitary landfilling 63
Scavengers 75
Schistosomiasis 30, 31
Sedimentation 35
Septic systems 28
Setback of house 50
Sewage treatment plant 64
Sewage waste water treatment
  aims of 66
  plant 66f
  process of 66
Sewer lines, leaks from 44
Shelter 13
Shrub layer 83
Slow sand 34
Small scale water purification 31
Snail 31
Social and economic 50
Socioculture environment 4
Soft water 25
Soil 88
  erosion 16
    control of 44
  pollution 43
    causes of 43
    control of 44
  waste 58
Solar energy 19
Solid waste 57
  management 59, 60*f*
    steps of 60
Sources, man-made 95
Space disposal 49
Species composition 75
Species, loss of useful 16
Specific conductivity 25
Spoiling birds' feathers 47
Sponge filter 24, 24*f*
Standard dry air 37
Standing crop 75
Standing state 75
State board, functions of 109
State Water Pollution Control Board, functions of 110
Stationary population 89
Stationary sources 37
Statutory towns 94
Storage 34
  tanks 28
Stratosphere 6
Sulfur dioxide 38
Sunlight, blocking out 47

Supernatant raw water 34
Surface runoff harvesting 22
Surface water pollution 27
Suspended solids 25

T

Taste, good 26
Temperate
  deciduous forests 83
  forests 82, 83
  grasslands 84
Temperature 25
  inequality of 52
Temporary deafness 42
Terrestrial biodiversity 101
Terrestrial biomes 71
Terrestrial ecosystem 82
Thermosphere 6
Threadworm 31
Tidal energy 19
Timber
  extraction 13
  wood 13
Total solids 25
Toxic
  chemical water pollution 27
  substances 9
Trachoma 30
Traditional agriculture 16
Transmission 5
Transmutation 49
Transport vehicles 41
Transportation 5, 23, 88
Trickling filter
  functioning of 68*f*
  principles of 68
Trophic level interaction 76
Trophic structure 75
Tropical forests 83
Tropical grasslands 84
Tropical rain forests 82
Troposphere 6
Typhoid 31

U

Unsanitary landfilling 64
Upper soil layer and vegetation, wastage of 15
Urban waste 44
Urbanization 92
  census of 94
Utilize environmentally friendly cleaning products 99

V

Varicella zoster 40
Ventilation 51
  standards of 52
  types of 52
Vermiculture 62
Viral 31

W

Waste 57
  management 57
    hierarchy of sustainable 60*f*
  recyclable 58
  recycling
    and reuse of 45
    of different material of 60
  specific source 58
  to energy combustion 63
  types of 57
Water 78
  (Prevention and Control of Pollution) Act 109
  chemical characteristics of 25
  color of 25
  conservation 28
    methods of 28
  cycle 79*f*
  energy 18
  hardness of 25
  large scale, purification of 33
  logging 17
  odor of 25
  pH value of 25
  physical characteristics of 22, 25
  pollution 14, 21, 26, 27
    categories of 27
    Cess Act 109
    sources of 27
  purification 31
  resources 13
    problems with 14
  sources of 22
    purification 28
  supply 51
  surface and ground 9
  taste of 25
  turbidity of 25

types of 24
use of 26
vapor 37
washed diseases 30
waste treatment 64
Water-based diseases 30
Waterbirds in chesapeake bay 77*f*
Waterborne diseases 29, 30
classification of 31*t*
Water-related diseases 30
Wave energy 19
Weil's disease 31
Western Ghats' biodiversity 102
Wet deposition 95
Wet phase 85
Wet scrubbers 39
Whooping cough 40
Wildlife
(protection) Act 111
Advisory Board, functions of 112
poaching of 103
Wind 52
power 18
Women education and employment 93
Wood 13
Worm composting 62